Satisfy a Woman

COSMO's
First-Ever
Book for
Guys

Satisfy a Woman

EVERY. SINGLE. TIME.

By the Editors of
COSMOPOLITAN

CFG COSMO FOR GUYS

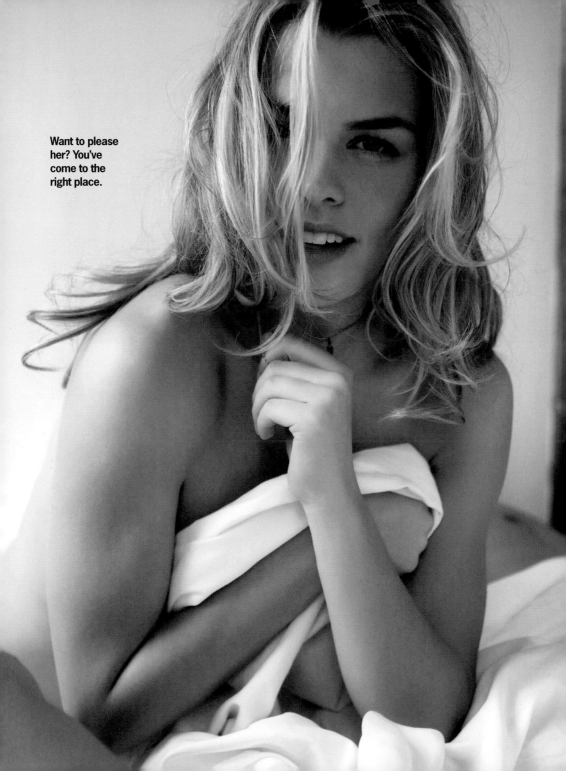

Want to please her? You've come to the right place.

Contents

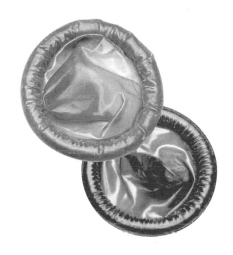

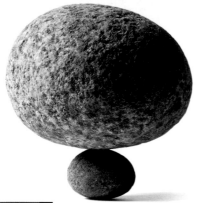

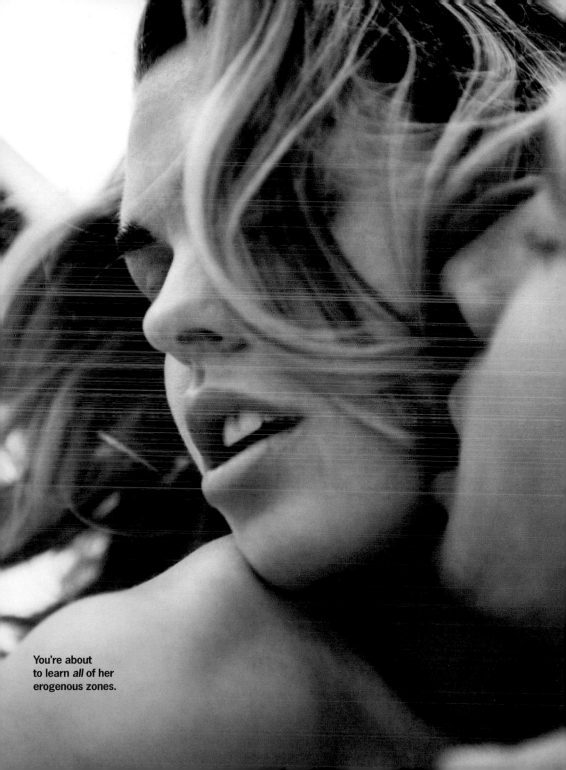

You're about
to learn *all* of her
erogenous zones.

Preface

The fact that you picked up this book means you're probably pretty damn good in bed. How do we know? (Don't worry, we haven't been talking to your former bedmates.) It's just that any guy who's curious about satisfying a woman clearly aims to please. The problem is that bringing her to orgasm is tricky business. No woman is the same, and we all need different things in order to reach that grand finale.

That's where Cosmo comes in. For years, guys have been telling us they peek at our magazine in hopes of finding out what women crave in bed. (And, yeah, we know the hot models and cleavage keep them coming back too.) Well, we decided to make it easier because women, after all, know best about what they want in the sack. Just like the title says, this book will arm you with all you need to know to satisfy a woman. We've packed these chapters so full of desire-inducing moves that you'll be sure to find something that'll work for the woman you're with.

We start with a step-by-step guide to her body. After that, we fill you in on the importance of lube (it makes helping her have an O so much easier!). Of course, we spend time on foreplay, suggesting moves that will leave her begging for more, and then break down how to actually give her that elusive orgasm. You'll also find a physiological explanation of what happens to her during sex, which will make it easier for you to understand her body and positions that make it simpler for her to finish. And if you run into any problems, we've got you covered with techniques to get her back on the road to O-Town.

So if you're ready to skyrocket your sexual IQ and bring her to the brink, go ahead and dig in.

—The Editors of Cosmo

CHAPTER 1

THE LAY OF HER LAND

To give her a mind-blowing orgasm, you've got to know more than just the precise moves to pull. In this chapter, you'll find all the info you need to know before you even walk into the bedroom, like where she's most sensitive and how to find that elusive G-spot. Read up and you'll be sure to earn an A the next time you're between the sheets with her.

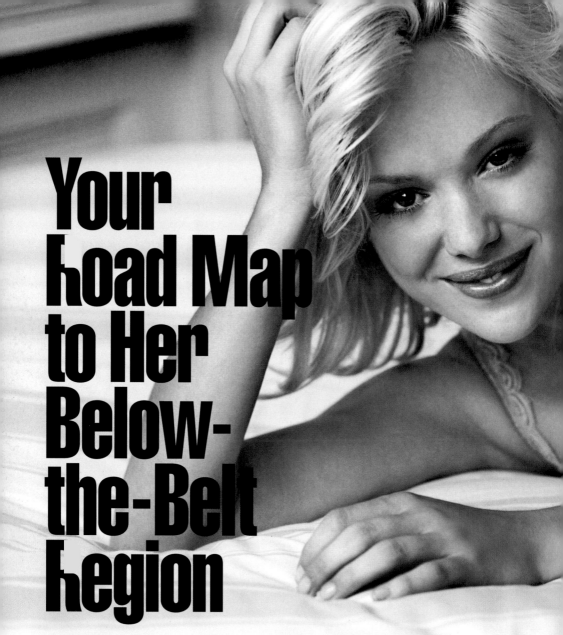

Your Road Map to Her Below-the-Belt Region

» Of course, you realize how important her down-there area is.
But to make sure you don't miss a single pleasure-packed spot,
here's everything you need to know for your trip south.

SATISFY A WOMAN—EVERY. SINGLE. TIME.

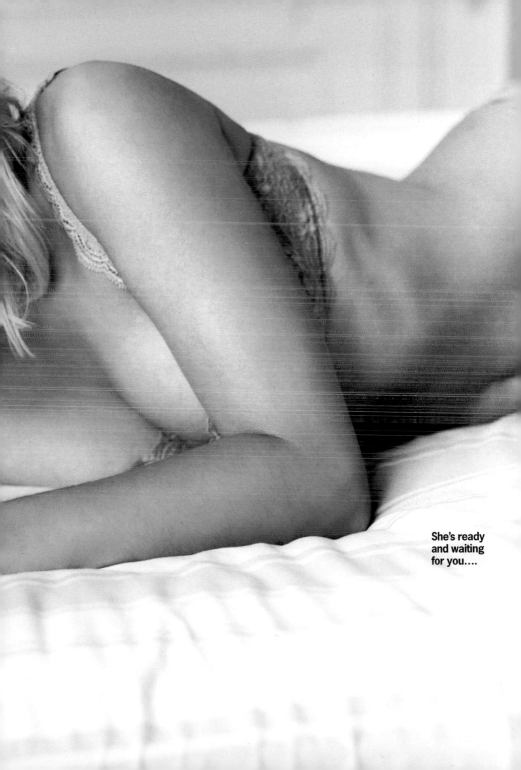

She's ready
and waiting
for you....

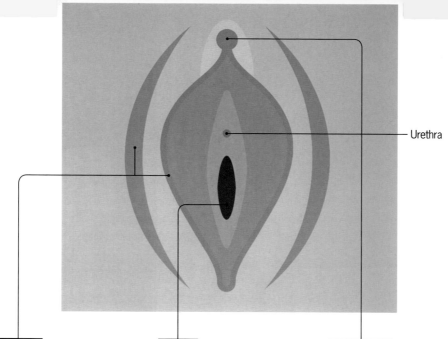

Urethra

LABIA

Women have inner and outer labia, which come in all different shapes and sizes. The lips on the outside protect the special parts inside (ahem, the clitoris), and they aren't super sensitive. However, the inner labia have lots of nerve endings, and it feels good for many women if you gently tug on them. They also connect to the clitoris, so touch her lips and she'll feel it there.

VAGINA

Many people incorrectly refer to the entire region between a woman's legs as the vagina. But the vagina is really just the internal area (where you penetrate). When a woman is aroused, her vaginal canal lengthens by about 4 inches to accommodate your shaft. The front wall has the most nerve endings, so any position that allows you to rub against that area—try missionary with a pillow under her butt—feels great for her.

CLITORIS

Consider this the MVP of her V team. How much attention you pay her clitoris determines whether she'll win—er, we mean orgasm. It is packed full of nerves and even gets erect when she's turned on. Oh, and that area is much bigger than it looks: There are nerve endings that extend several inches under the labia and toward the vaginal opening. You may not see the little love button when you first look

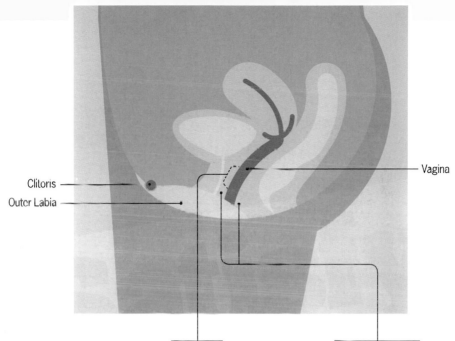

Clitoris

Outer Labia

Vagina

G-SPOT

PC MUSCLES

down there—a hood of skin protects it, since it's incredibly sensitive. The key is to start off with a light touch, as using too much pressure too soon can be painful for her.

You can't see it. You can't feel it. But ask most women and they'll tell you that this nerve-packed area exists. Where can you find it? About 2 inches inside her vagina on the front side (toward the belly button). Rub your penis or fingers over it and you'll send her spiraling out control with desire. Flip to page 68 for precise G-spot moves.

Also known as the pubococcygeus (don't ask us how that's pronounced!), these are the muscles in her pelvic floor that help her hold in pee. If she squeezes them during sex (known as doing Kegels), it makes a tighter fit for you and sends feel-good spasms through her body.

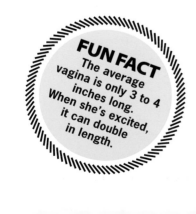

FUN FACT
The average vagina is only 3 to 4 inches long. When she's excited, it can double in length.

SOURCE: MARY JANE MINKIN, MD, CLINICAL PROFESSOR OF OB-GYN AT THE YALE UNIVERSITY SCHOOL OF MEDICINE

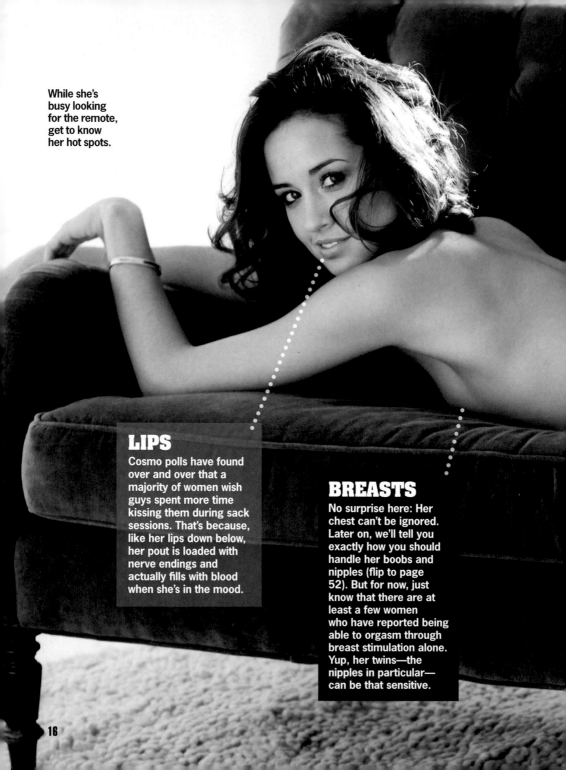

While she's busy looking for the remote, get to know her hot spots.

LIPS

Cosmo polls have found over and over that a majority of women wish guys spent more time kissing them during sack sessions. That's because, like her lips down below, her pout is loaded with nerve endings and actually fills with blood when she's in the mood.

BREASTS

No surprise here: Her chest can't be ignored. Later on, we'll tell you exactly how you should handle her boobs and nipples (flip to page 52). But for now, just know that there are at least a few women who have reported being able to orgasm through breast stimulation alone. Yup, her twins—the nipples in particular—can be that sensitive.

Her Other Sexy Parts...

>> Men who focus only on her down-there bits are okay in bed. But it's the guys who tease and tantalize other erogenous zones that are remembered as rock stars in the sack. If you want to be that guy (and why wouldn't you?!), consider these your must-visit areas.

BUTT

Whether you prefer some junk in the trunk or an itty-bitty booty, the ass is a big-time erogenous zone. It's home to the largest muscle in the body, so kneading it while you're making out will relax her into a more sensual state. (Or give it a light slap.) When she's turned on, her body releases feel-good chemicals called endorphins, which make those pats feel pretty damn good.

FEET

Each foot has a large concentration of nerve endings—particularly in the toes and the soles. If sucking her toes isn't your thing, a firm-pressure massage will have the exact same effect.

MORE >>

Her inner thighs are a minefield of sensitivity.

EARS

Two reasons these are such hot spots: First, the lobes are incredibly responsive to touch, so sucking on them feels *ahhh*mazing for her. Second, when women hear what naughty things you want to do to them, it puts their arousal into overdrive. Some experts say that the simple act of talking dirty can prime her for sex just as well as physical touch can.

NECK

Her skin is very thin here, making it ultra sensitive, so light kisses, licks, and nibbles are almost always welcome. Or send shivers down her spine by licking from her collarbone to her ear and then lightly blowing on the area. The combo of your warm tongue and cool breath will arouse the hell out of her.

INNER THIGHS

The insides of her upper legs often get neglected due to their proximity to the promise land. You guys probably figure, *Why touch there when I can touch somewhere even better?* But you're missing a big opportunity, because the inner thighs are a minefield of sensitivity. Even the lightest strokes carry pleasure straight to her groin.

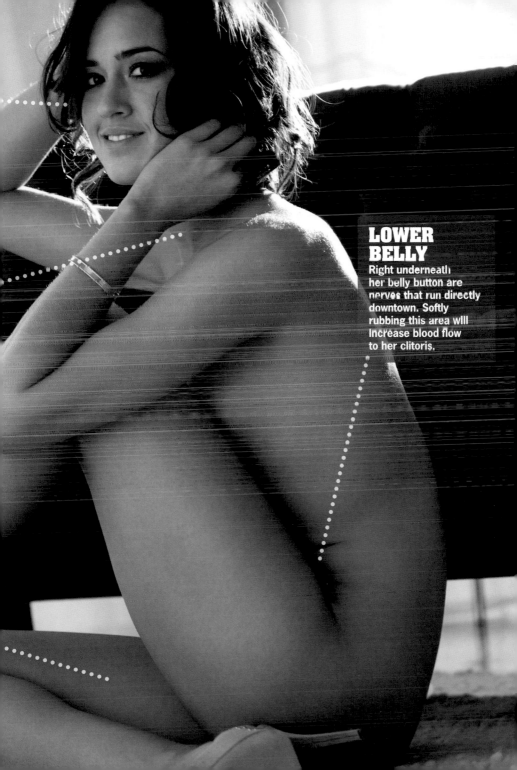

LOWER BELLY

Right underneath her belly button are nerves that run directly downtown. Softly rubbing this area will increase blood flow to her clitoris.

CHAPTER 2

MAKE LIKE A BOY SCOUT

(and Always Be Prepared)

Now that you're a pro at navigating her bod, there are just a few more things you should know so you're totally equipped to blow her mind. From condoms to lube to manscaping, we have all the info you need.

Rubber Rules

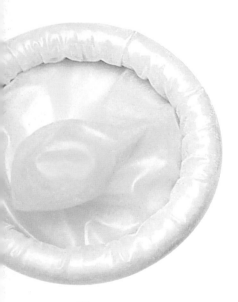

>> We're not your mother, so we won't lecture you on why condoms are important. After all, we assume you don't want an STD or unwanted pregnancy and you're using them as necessary. And one thing you may not realize is that when you whip one out, it instantly puts a chick's mind at ease. She knows that you're both being responsible and that she doesn't have to worry, which lets her enjoy the moment even more. When it does come time to roll one on, there is a certain etiquette you should follow.

Slip one on and you're good to go.

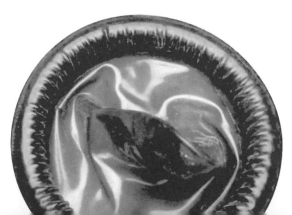

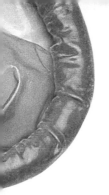

1
Don't expect her to have a condom.
You're the one who will be wearing the prophylactic, so you should be the one who has it. Think of it this way: She doesn't make you pick up her birth-control pills, so you shouldn't assume she'll supply your condoms.

2
Never pull it out of your wallet.
Yes, it's convenient, but experts say that can actually weaken the effectiveness because the package can get bent and torn. (Side note: It also makes you look like a movie cliché, and she'll think it's a little lame.)

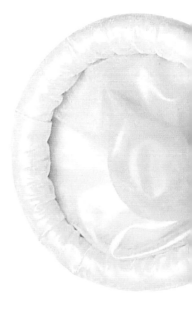

3
Know how to put it on.
When it takes a ton of time to sheath your member, it can be a buzzkill. Hell, practice at home if you must—for both of your sakes. Here's a refresher course: Hold the condom in one hand and your penis in the other. Pinch the tip, and then unroll the condom down the length of your shaft.

4
If you throw the used rubber on her floor afterward, she may kick your ass.
Seriously, she doesn't want to have to pick it up, and she certainly doesn't want to have to Google "How to get semen out of a rug."

Since you'll be the one wearing the thing, you should have it on you.

Buy the Right Condoms

>> If you've been in the rubber aisle recently, you've probably thought, *What the hell are all these different kinds?!* Don't worry, we've got your back. Here's the lowdown on each type.

THE MATERIALS

LATEX

These are made from a type of rubber and are the most common and readily available; they also tend to be cheaper. According to the American Academy of Allergy, Asthma, and Immunology, up to 6 percent of people are allergic to latex, so if either of you gets itchy, red, or puffy afterward, you may want to talk to a doctor about a possible allergy.

POLYURETHANE

This type of love glove is made out of plastic. They are thinner and slightly less constricting than their latex counterparts. Keep this in mind: Studies have shown that polyurethane condoms break more often than latex ones do.

THE STYLES AND SHAPES

RIBBED

These guys have a bumpy texture built in, which is supposed to stimulate the nerve endings in the vaginal walls. But some women say they can't really feel it.

POUCHED

A sheath like this has "pockets" near the tip or on the sides, so it fits more loosely in those areas, increasing friction and sensitivity for you.

ULTRATHIN

The thinner the condom, the more you'll both feel. Just be extra careful when you're using these, as they are more delicate than regular ones.

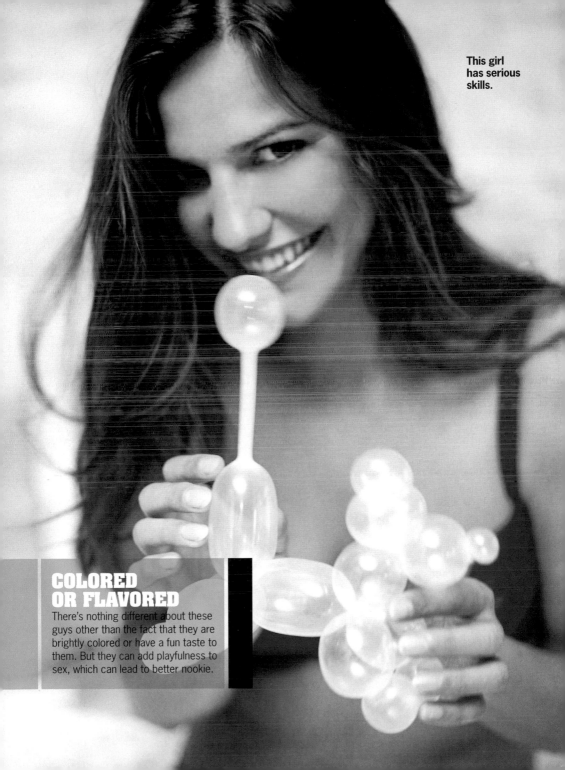

This girl has serious skills.

COLORED OR FLAVORED

There's nothing different about these guys other than the fact that they are brightly colored or have a fun taste to them. But they can add playfulness to sex, which can lead to better nookie.

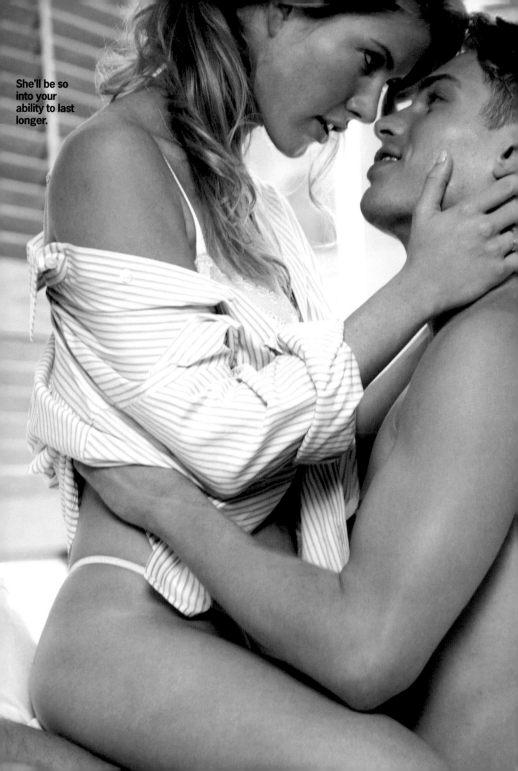

She'll be so into your ability to last longer.

Condom Problem Solving

>> It can be awkward, annoying, or flat-out freaky when something goes wrong with your protection. To help put your mind at ease, we've got info and tips on the most common mishaps.

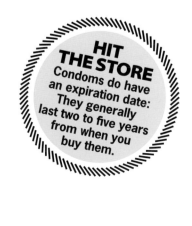

HIT THE STORE
Condoms do have an expiration date: They generally last two to five years from when you buy them.

One of You Has a Latex Allergy

If either of you feels itching or burning when using a condom, try a polyurethane option, and avoid any with spermicide, which can cause irritation even if you aren't allergic.

They Make You Lose Your Erection

Try a cock ring. It's a small plastic band you place around the base of your shaft and around your testicles that keeps the blood supply from draining from your penis

It Feels Too Tight

Put a drop of lube in the tip before rolling it on. It'll help the rubber glide and move as you thrust. If that doesn't work, try a condom made for larger penises (like Trojan Magnum).

You Can't Last Quite as Long as She Wants

Check out Durex Performax or Trojan Extended Pleasure condoms. Both are lubricated with a slight numbing agent that'll keep you going longer.

The Rubber Breaks

Both of you should wash yourselves with soap and water. Then see a doctor as soon as you can to be tested for STDs. If she's not on birth-control pills, she should get emergency contraception (called Plan B One-Step) from a local pharmacy within 72 hours.

The Lube Lowdown

>> This sexy little bottle can take you from being a great lover to being the best-sex-of-her-life kind of guy. Being extralubricated not only lets you do more serious thrusting—it also helps her finish with a bang. "The wetter a woman is, the easier it is for a man to vary the speed and thrust continuously," says sex therapist Debra Macleod, coauthor of *Lube Jobs: A Woman's Guide to Great Maintenance Sex.* "And that combination can build the sexual tension and bring her to orgasm." But just because wetter is better doesn't mean you should use a whole bottle. A dime-size dollop will make things plenty slippery. As for what kind you should use, well, it's really up to you. There are tons of varieties available—here are three you should be familiar with.

WATER-BASED

This is the most common lube on store shelves. It's smooth and slick, and it feels most like her natural lubricant. Since it's water-soluble, her skin will naturally start to absorb it. That means you may need to reapply if you're having a marathon sack session.

SILICONE-BASED

This is the Energizer Bunny of lubes—it never dies! Meaning, it simply never dries out, so there's never a need to reapply. Of course, that staying power comes with a downside: It can be a bit messy to clean up. Experts suggest you save this type for the shower.

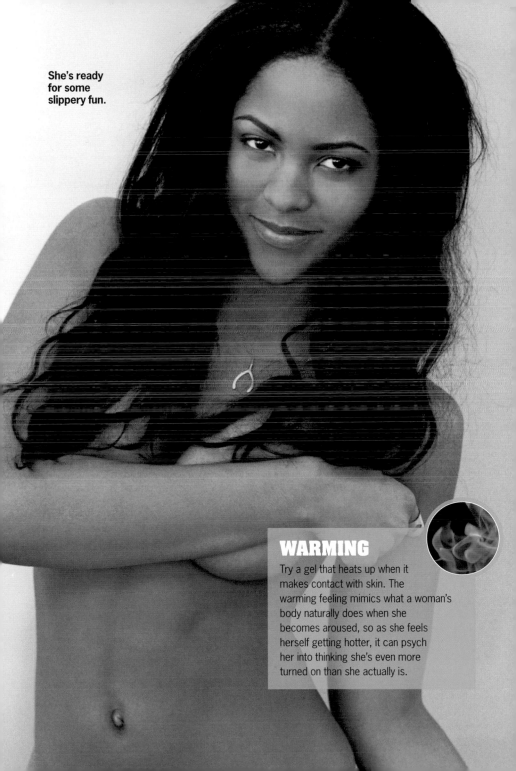

She's ready
for some
slippery fun.

WARMING

Try a gel that heats up when it makes contact with skin. The warming feeling mimics what a woman's body naturally does when she becomes aroused, so as she feels herself getting hotter, it can psych her into thinking she's even more turned on than she actually is.

Do a Little Man Prep

>> Before we tell you how to get her primed for the main event, let us fill you in on the prep work she expects you to have done to yourself. Following these grooming rules will ensure she doesn't run out of the room before you have a chance to slip between the sheets.

1 SMELL GOOD DOWN THERE

We know it's natural to sweat throughout the course of the day. But if your junk smells even the slightest bit funky, no chick is going to go near it. Luckily, you don't have to take a full shower every time you want to get laid; just wipe yourself down quickly with a washcloth before the action begins.

2 KEEP YOUR BEARD SOFT

She loves to kiss, but when your facial hair scratches the hell out of her face, she'll be in pain and the mood will go from hot to cold, fast. Plus, if it bothers her face, it's sure to irritate other, more sensitive areas. In your morning shower, rub a little conditioner onto your scruff, then rinse it off. This softens your fuzz just enough so that it won't do any lasting damage.

3 DON'T BE AFRAID TO MANSCAPE

If a girl had a '70s-style bush, you might be a tad weirded out. Well, she'll feel the same way if you're rockin' similarly untamed pubes. But that doesn't mean you have to go bare. In fact, 73 percent of women say they prefer a neat trim to no hair at all (use manicure scissors to fix up). Bonus: The less hair down there, the bigger your package looks.

SATISFY A WOMAN—EVERY. SINGLE. TIME.

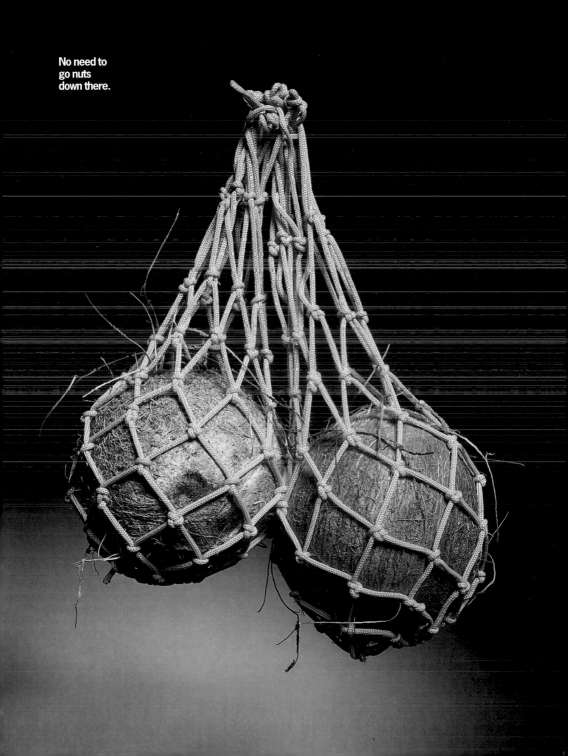

No need to
go nuts
down there.

CHAPTER 3

GET HER FIRED UP

She's not a TV dinner. Meaning, you can't pop her in the microwave on high for a few minutes and expect her to be ready to go— at least not if you want to be unforgettable in the sack. "Men get an erection and want action," says sex therapist Carole Altman, PhD. "Women need to be stimulated and teased for a while before their body is ready." But we promise, putting in the effort will have a big payoff for you too. The more turned on she is, the more into things she'll be, making the hookup way more exciting for you both. Flip the page for all the presex moves you should have in your arsenal.

»

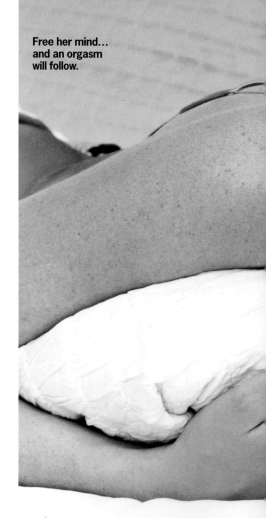

Free her mind…
and an orgasm
will follow.

Seduce Her... Brain

>> There's one major difference between men and women when it comes to crossing the finish line: While you can orgasm based purely on physical sensations, most females can't. "Women tend to be more affected by extraneous thoughts during sex," says Ian Kerner, PhD, author of *She Comes First*. "So if she has a lot going on at work or is stressed out, she may not be able to let her mind go enough to orgasm." That means that even if your moves are amazing, she still might have a hard time climaxing. But you can fight off those external thoughts by getting her to stay in the moment. Here are four easy ways to keep her brain in the game.

1 Clean up a bit.
Mess stresses out a lot of women, and it may make her think about cleaning while you're touching her. Not exactly hot. If the room's tidy, she'll be able to focus.

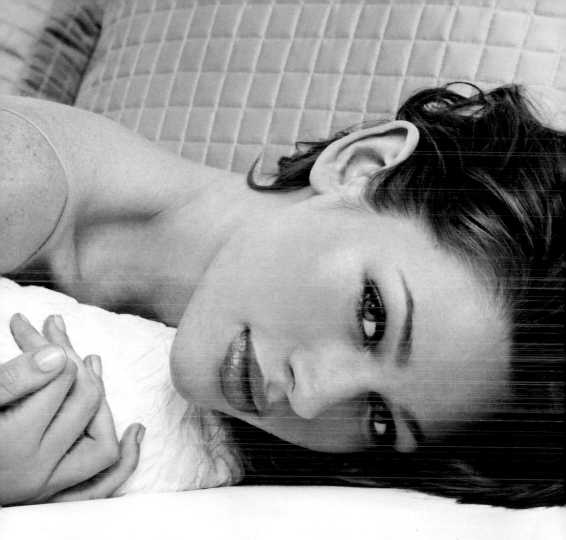

2 Turn off your phone.
If she hears a ring or a text-message notification, she'll be wondering who it is instead of thinking about your killer moves.

3 Extend foreplay.
By going just five minutes longer, you give her even more opportunity to get into it, and she'll be likelier to forget about everything else that happened during the day.

4 Keep telling her the dirty things you're going to do next.
Having an X-rated convo forces her to focus on what's going on right then.

Turn Her On All Day Long

>> Foreplay doesn't have to start right before sex. In fact, putting in a little work throughout the day can really help her later on. See, studies show that when a woman has been on a slow simmer (meaning she's been turned on for a while), it's easier for her to orgasm. Do these simple things and she'll be raring to go by the time you climb into bed.

When she walks

through the front door, give her a long hug, making sure your hand lingers on her ass for a few seconds.

Before she leaves

for work, tell her how good her butt looks in the skirt she's wearing.

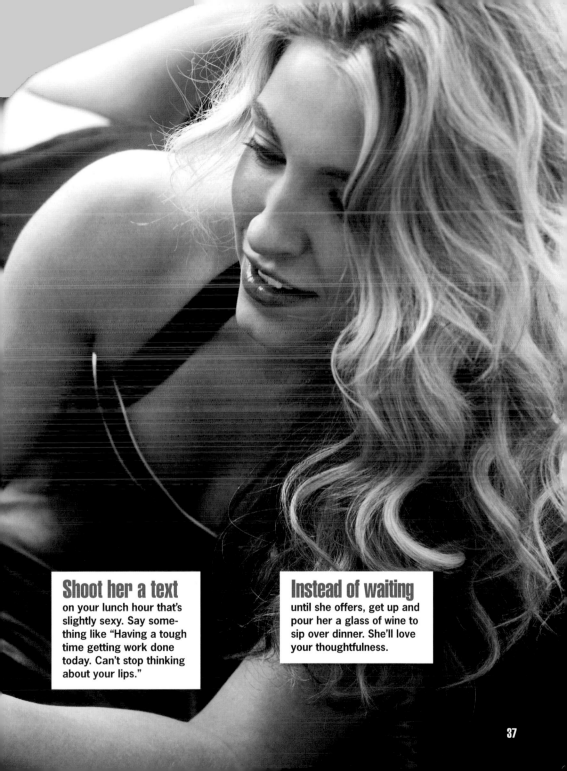

Shoot her a text

on your lunch hour that's slightly sexy. Say something like "Having a tough time getting work done today. Can't stop thinking about your lips."

Instead of waiting

until she offers, get up and pour her a glass of wine to sip over dinner. She'll love your thoughtfulness.

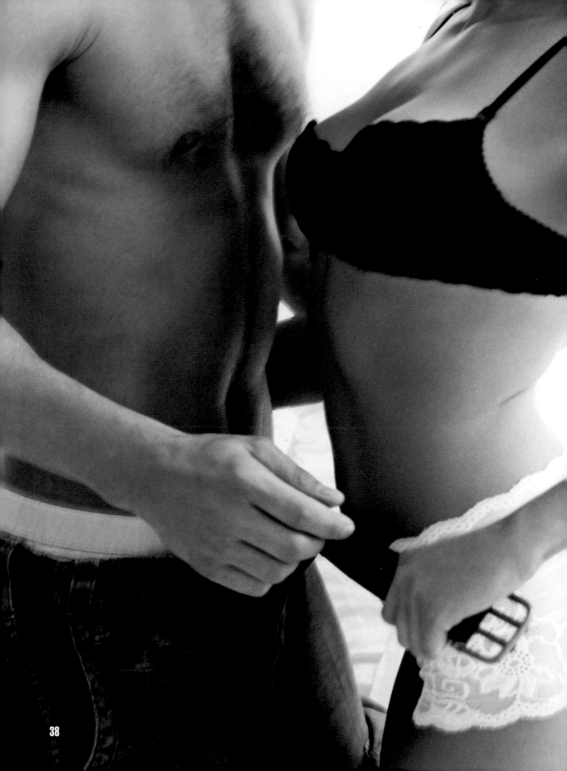

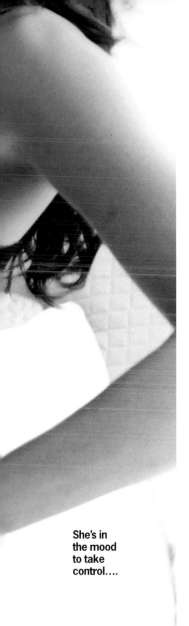

She's in the mood to take control....

Predict the Sex She's Craving

>> The next step that will take you from good to great is figuring out the type of nookie she's craving. Asking her flat out what she's looking for kind of kills the mood. Fortunately, women send signs. Know how to read them and she'll think you're a genius.

SIGNALS SHE'S SENDING:

- While watching TV, she uses a light touch to stroke your arm *uuup* and *dooown*.
- She gives you a deep kiss with a little tongue... but not too much.
- There's a candle lit by her bedside table or she's thrown a scarf over her lamp.
- Her voice is a little huskier than usual.

HER MOOD: Sensual and soft

SIGNALS SHE'S SENDING:

- She nips at your bottom lip while you're kissing.
- She puts on sexy music that has a lot of electric guitar and drums in it.
- Her nails dig lightly into your back as you suck on her neck.
- She gives some direct orders ("Give me a massage," "Come into the bedroom now," etc.).

HER MOOD: Rough-and-tumble

If you know how to read the signals she sends, you'll figure out exactly what she's looking for.

SIGNALS SHE'S SENDING:

- She's in the middle of another task—like reading a book or cooking dinner—but still sends you major flirt signals.
- You're in bed together, and she tells you how tired she is while rubbing her feet all along your leg.
- When you go to touch her down below, she pushes your hand away and unbuttons your pants.

HER MOOD: Quick and easy

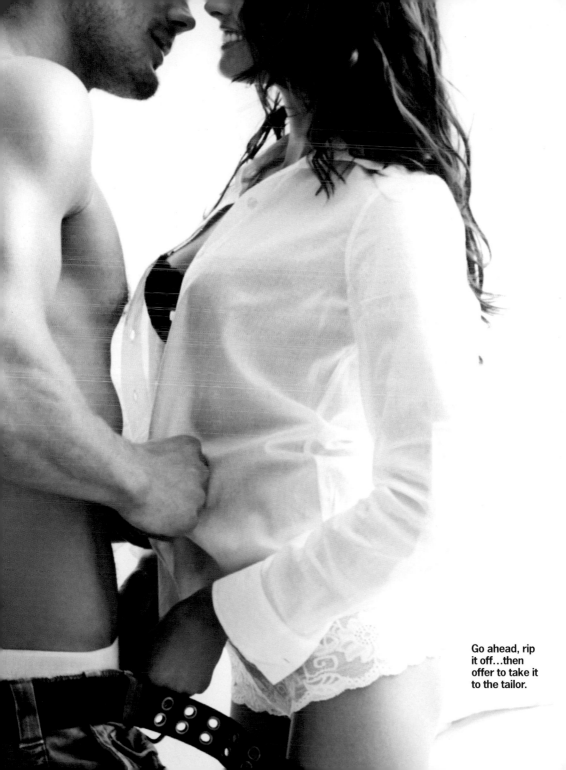

Go ahead, rip it off…then offer to take it to the tailor.

Get Her in the Mood

>> Those sex scenes in movies where there are rose petals strewn everywhere and a gajillion candles lit? So freakin' cheesy. Most women don't want that stuff. But to be memorable, you do need to set the mood a little. So you don't cross that schmaltz-factor line, we tell you what's just enough romance and what's way too much.

JUST ENOUGH	WAY TOO FAR
Playing Spanish guitar music or a cool new R&B song in the background	Blasting Barry White or Marvin Gaye when she walks in the room
Lighting a single scented candle on your nightstand	Covering every available surface with tea lights—lame *and* a fire hazard!
Splurging on 100 percent cotton sheets with a high thread count so your bed is extra inviting	Satin sheets. Just don't go there.
Leaving a jar of chocolate body paint somewhere in the bedroom for her to find	Force-feeding her chocolate-covered strawberries right before you want her to get naked

Candles and a warm bath? Perfect. But add a million rose petals and you've gone cliché.

Set this scene for her and she's all yours.

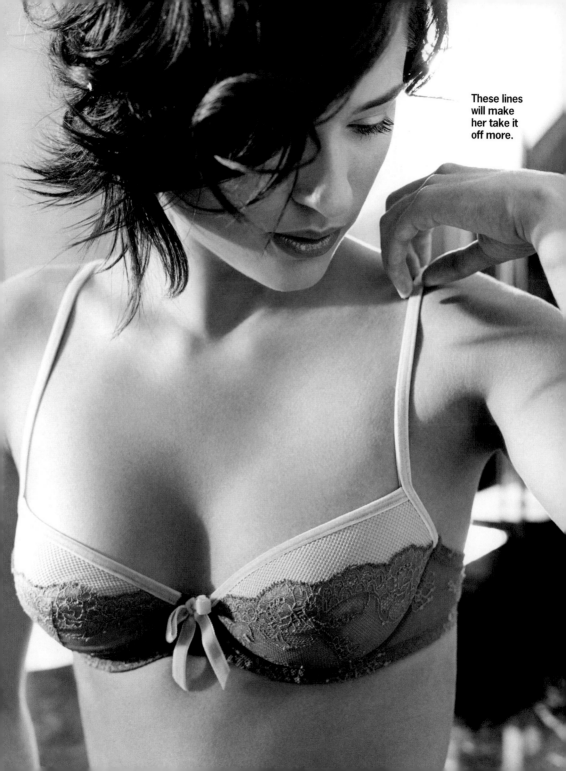

These lines
will make
her take it
off more.

Make Her Feel Sexy Naked

>> Almost every woman, even the ridiculously hot ones, feels a little self-conscious naked. Hey, it's a vulnerable state to be in! "While it is natural for a woman to do this, you really don't want her stressing about her body in bed," says sexologist Patricia Love, EdD. "The more she worries, the less carefree and fun she'll be to sleep with." One way to make her feel great about how she looks sans clothing is to randomly give her little compliments. Tell her any of these and she'll appreciate her body even more.

"Are you working out more? You've been looking even hotter than usual."

"Man, you look incredible in that bra."

"You have no idea how often I think about how lucky I am to be with a girl with such a bangin' body."

"You look so good when you're on top of me."

"Sometimes I catch other guys checking you out as you walk by. I know I should be mad at them, but I can't really blame them."

"Please bend over again, your ass looks *sooo* good when you do that."

"Do you know how perfect your breasts are? Seriously, they're the best I've ever seen."

Give Her an Erotic Massage

>> There's something about a rubdown that makes a woman feel incredibly sexy—between being touched all over and the relaxed feeling, how could she not? So if you give her one presex, she'll be putty in your hands.

1 Before you strip her down, make sure the room is warm enough that she'll be comfortable (a cold temperature will just make her tense up and shiver). Once she's lying facedown on the bed, warm up some lotion or massage oil between your hands. Since you'll be having sex later, make sure the product is water-based (so it won't affect the condom).

2 Start rubbing her shoulders lightly, using your thumbs to gently massage her shoulder blades. Then trail your fingers down to her lower back. This is where women store most of their stress, so spend a little longer here. Use your knuckles to gently knead the area. Finally, run your fingers along her backside, and tickle where her booty meets her thighs (it's sensitive there; this will send tingles all over).

3 Since the point of this particular massage is to turn her on, not make her fall asleep, make sure you incorporate some light kisses and licks along the way to keep her turned on and stimulated.

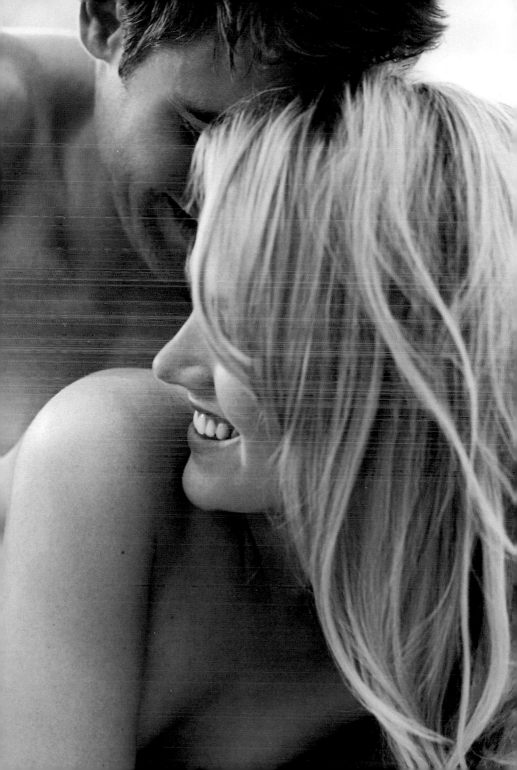

Yup, You Gotta Kiss Her

>> Think back to junior high, when pretty much all you did was make out. Remember how exciting it was? Then you hit second and third bases, and kissing seemed less thrilling. Here's the thing: Women love it and wish you'd do more of it. "There are tons of nerve endings in your lips that stimulate desire," says Krista Bloom, PhD, author of *The Ultimate Compatibility Quiz.* "Locking lips before intercourse can be extremely arousing and satisfying." On top of that, your saliva carries testosterone, and when you transfer that to her, it actually increases her sex drive. The trick is to start softly and then get more aggressive. Try these tips to really get her going.

START SLOWLY...

Warm her up before launching into full-throttle passion. "Part of what excites her is the slow, steady build of a kiss," says Bloom. "So it's much more erotic to begin with light smooches."

Give her little pecks all over her cheeks and neck—totally avoiding her mouth. Once you can sense her aching for lip-on-lip action, trace the outline of her mouth with your tongue.

Move on to open-mouth kissing, but keep the anticipation building by not using your tongue.

Get playful and softly tug on her bottom lip with your teeth.

NOW TURN UP THE HEAT

After keeping it tame for a while, it's time to accelerate things. "Passionate kisses elevate your blood pressure and cause your heart to beat faster, getting you more excited and making it easier for her to reach orgasm," says certified sexologist Ava Cadell, PhD. So stoke that fire.

Vary the intensity of lip-locks. Give her a soft French kiss, and then surprise her by pressing your lips against hers—hard and aggressively.

Take her tongue into your mouth, and gently suck.

Swirl your tongue around hers in a circular motion—it creates a new sensation that's surprising and fun.

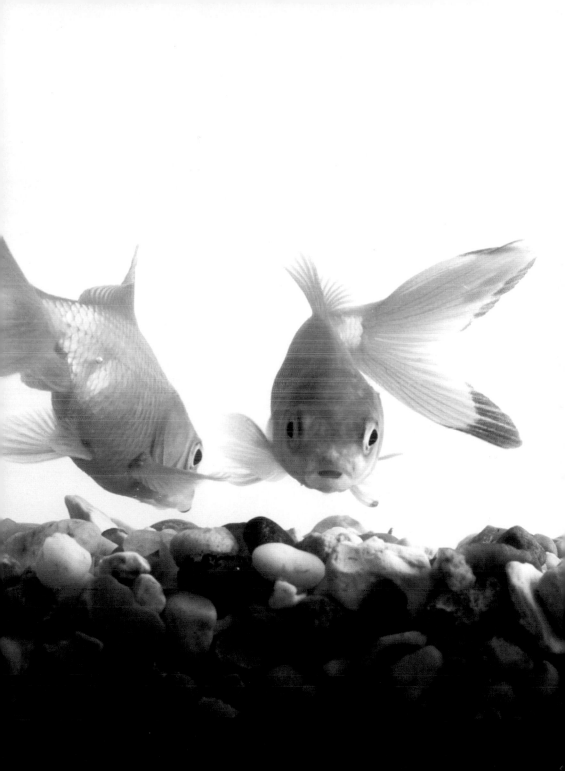

Lots of tongue
is A-OK with
some chicks.

> **" It's pretty simple:** Reach down and grab my ass while your mouth is on mine. It is animalistic and revs me up."
> —*Jenn, 30*

> **" I prefer romantic kisses,** so when a man looks deeply into my eyes beforehand, it makes the entire experience feel more sensual."
> —*Kristen, 24*

Women's Pucker Confessions

» Real chicks open up about even more smooch moves that get them going.

> **" One thing that sends me** over the edge is when a guy gently grabs the hair at the back of my neck and lightly pulls it to angle my face up to his before swooping in for a lip-lock."
> —*Sarah, 26*

> **" I love when a** guy presses me up against a wall while laying one on me. It makes it feel even more intense."
> —*Dina, 32*

> **" When a guy talks to me** in between kisses, it can make it so much hotter. All he has to do is pull back every once in a while and tell me how much he likes me."
> —*Jessie, 23*

Handle Her Breasts

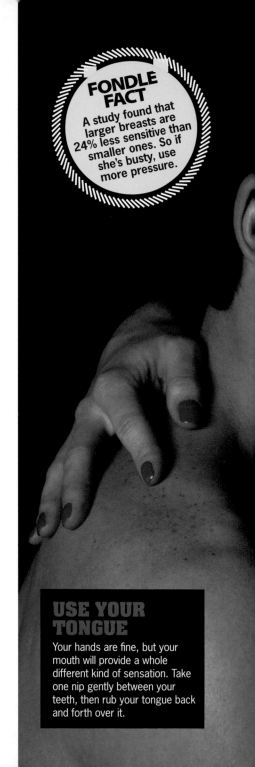

>> We have no doubt that you love boobs. And we're glad, because the more attention you pay to them, the more hyped up most women get. But it takes the right kind of touching, and unfortunately, many men don't do it right. We often hear from readers who say their guy either manhandles their pair or treats them as if they were made of glass. Try these moves and she'll have zero complaints.

VENTURE OUTSIDE THE NIPPLES

Yes, the nipples are the most sensitive. But that doesn't mean you should focus only there. In fact, if the sole places you touch are those little nubs, she might grow desensitized. Lightly run your fingertips in circles, starting on the outer edge of her breasts and zeroing in until you reach the areolae.

USE YOUR TONGUE

Your hands are fine, but your mouth will provide a whole different kind of sensation. Take one nip gently between your teeth, then rub your tongue back and forth over it.

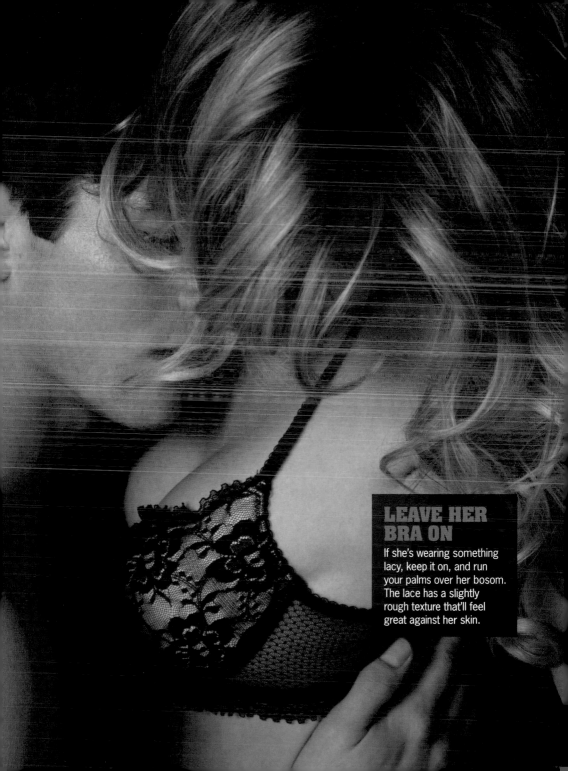

LEAVE HER BRA ON

If she's wearing something lacy, keep it on, and run your palms over her bosom. The lace has a slightly rough texture that'll feel great against her skin.

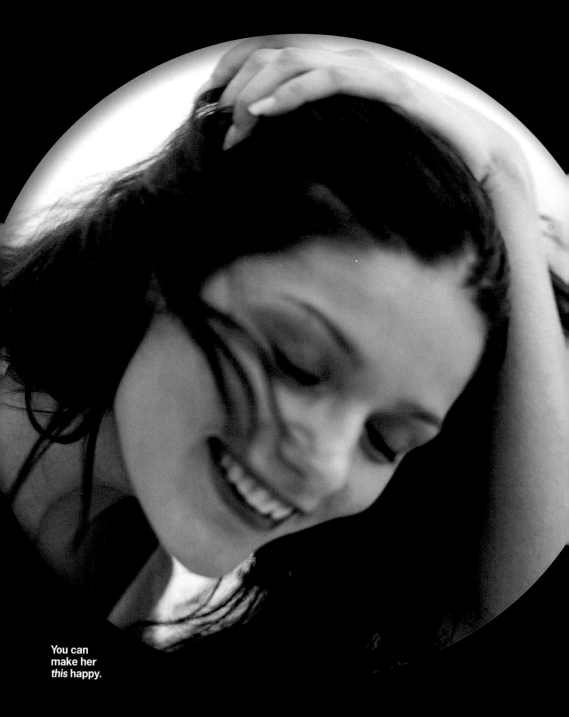

You can
make her
this happy.

Her Masturbation Secrets

>> Solo sex is a tricky subject when it comes to women — studies show that 92 percent of them do it, but many don't feel comfortable talking about it. You should not only get her to chat about it with you—you should ask her to masturbate in front of you. See, she knows her body best and can get herself off quickly and easily. So if you're able to watch, you'll pick up invaluable info. "Tell your girlfriend or wife that you can think of nothing more arousing than watching her pleasure herself," says sex therapist Judith Seifer, PhD. "If she feels weird about it, say you'll help her out by touching her in other places." It may take her a while to feel okay about doing it in front of you, but if you occasionally mention how fired up it would get you, she might want to try it. In the meantime, learn from what real women told us about their self-lovin' tactics.

A Sensual Mood

"I make touching myself an event. I put on lotion, light some candles, and turn on music. It makes me feel taken care of and extra sexy."
—*Gabrielle, 24*

A Little Warm-Up

"I run my fingers from my belly button to my nipples over and over. Warming up the rest of my body before concentrating on my clitoris helps big time." —*Melanie, 34*

Not the Typical Place

"I like to pleasure myself in the bathtub. The warm water is relaxing and sensual." —*Erin, 26*

Switching Up the Moves

"I rub my clitoris slowly and then speed up. Then I pull back and do it again, more leisurely. I go back and forth until I finally finish." —*Diane, 31*

Adding Gadgets

"I use a vibrator on my clitoris to really rev me up. Then when I'm close, I'll stick a finger inside myself. That almost always makes me orgasm." —*Laney, 29*

Hands-On Fun

>> Would you like it if she simply moved her hands up and down your shaft? Hell no! Well, women like more intricate palm moves too. These tricks are sure to please. Oh, and you should know that some women have a hard time climaxing during sex and can reach that point only with manual or oral—making these moves even more important.

He's about to attempt the heel feel.

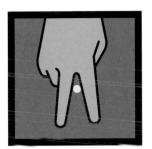

THE V JOB

Make a V with your middle and pointer fingers, and place them on either side of her clitoris. Then move your digits up and down. This indirect touch lets a slow fire build.

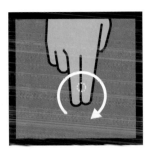

AROUND THE WORLD

Keeping your pointer and middle fingers together, place them directly over that little ecstasy button and move them in a circular motion. Start slowly, and pick up speed.

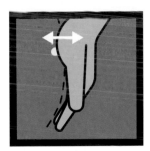

THE HEEL FEEL

Place the heel of your hand over her clitoris, and alternate pushing into it and releasing it. Because your palm is wide, it distributes the pressure and won't put too much on that supersensitive spot.

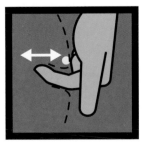

THE COME HITHER

Insert your finger inside her, and rub the area 2 inches up on the inside—that's about where her G-spot is. Then make a "come hither" motion. By getting her G-spot into the game early on, you ensure that it's even more sensitive later.

Oral Tricks & Tips

THE WINDSHIELD WIPER

Point your tongue, and move it in an arc up and over her clitoris. Keep repeating until she's squirming with desire.

THE SNAKE

Place your mouth right over the opening of her vagina. Then stick out your tongue so it's thin and firm, and flick it in and out of her, like a snake. The entrance of her V zone is where most of the nerves are, so it'll feel extra good.

THE SENSUAL SUCK

Stick out your lips (as if you were going to give her a peck), place them around her clitoris, and gently suck. Instead of providing direct stimulation, this puts heavenly pressure on that sexy spot.

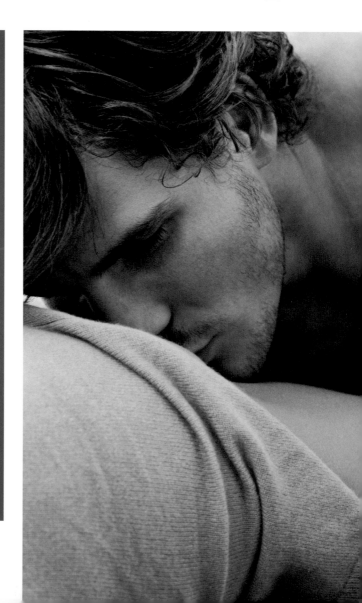

Never underestimate the power of your tongue. Whether you want to get her primed or bring her all the way to orgasm, these mouth maneuvers will seriously wow her… and probably make her scream your name.

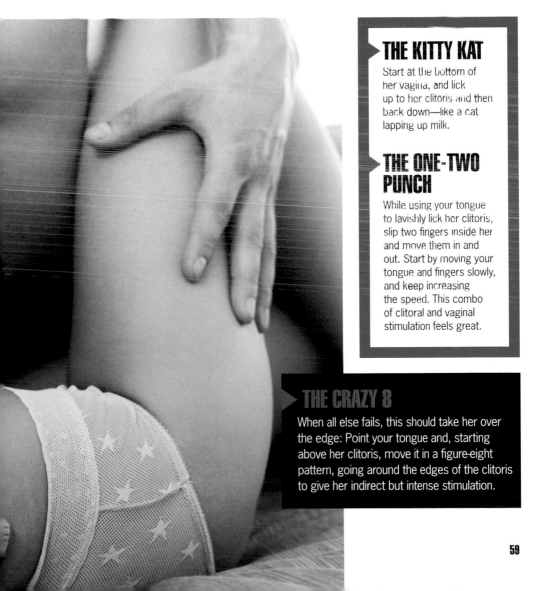

THE KITTY KAT

Start at the bottom of her vagina, and lick up to her clitoris and then back down—like a cat lapping up milk.

THE ONE-TWO PUNCH

While using your tongue to lavishly lick her clitoris, slip two fingers inside her and move them in and out. Start by moving your tongue and fingers slowly, and keep increasing the speed. This combo of clitoral and vaginal stimulation feels great.

THE CRAZY 8

When all else fails, this should take her over the edge: Point your tongue and, starting above her clitoris, move it in a figure-eight pattern, going around the edges of the clitoris to give her indirect but intense stimulation.

The Art of 69

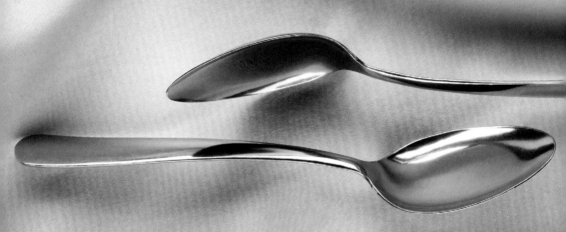

>> There's nothing better than both of you getting intense pleasure at the exact same time, and 69 allows you to do just that. You can make her squirm with passion, and the fact that she can do the same to you simultaneously makes it even more fun. Now, literally going head to toe requires a bit of coordination, but it's *sooo* worth it. Here are the easiest 69ing positions.

HER ON TOP

Have her straddle your upper chest so she's facing away from you. Guide her hips back so your mouth can easily reach her. Tell her if she rounds her back, it'll make it even easier for you.

SIDE BY SIDE

Both of you should lie on your sides, with your head near her crotch. Bend her top leg back so her knee is in the air and her foot is flat on the bed behind her other knee. This will open her up for you, making it easier for you to go to town with your tongue.

YOU ON TOP

Kneel over her face, then get down on your elbows so that your hips are still elevated and your face is between her legs. This requires a bit more strength on your part but gives her great access to your shaft. Just be sure not to thrust—you don't want to choke her, after all!

She Hates It When...

Now that we've told you what she'll like, real women chime in on what they *don't* like during foreplay.

"Men shouldn't be afraid to get a little rough during foreplay. Nothing turns me on more than when a guy uses his teeth to lightly graze my nipples, moves me where he wants me to be, or firmly grabs my ass as wo kiss."
—Sara, 24

"When a guy kisses a trail from my breasts to my belly button, I go crazy. It's sensual, romantic, and hot."
—Deb, 26

She Loves It When...

And of course, we wouldn't want to end on a negative note. Here's what drives some women crazy in the beginning stages of a hookup.

"I like it when a guy doesn't take himself too seriously in the bedroom. If he turns on fun, upbeat music, it excites me because I know he's looking for a good time and isn't going to be uptight in bed."
—Sue, 30

"I could almost orgasm from neck kissing alone. Seriously, the way to get me really wet is to spend a lot of time kissing there. Then switch it up and lick a trail from the bottom of my ear to my collarbone and back. It feels incredibly sensual, and that is such a sensitive spot that makes me tingle all over."
—Carrie, 28

"There's something erotic about a man undressing me—taking off my clothes one item at a time, stopping to kiss me deeply every once in a while."
—Lauren, 25

CHAPTER 4

TAKE HER TO O-TOWN

Drumroll, please…welcome to the main event! Now that you know how to get her primed, you're ready for what it takes to make you truly unforgettable: giving her an orgasm. In this chapter, you'll find all the info you'll need to do the job— positions that wow, the different kinds of climaxes you can give her, and more.

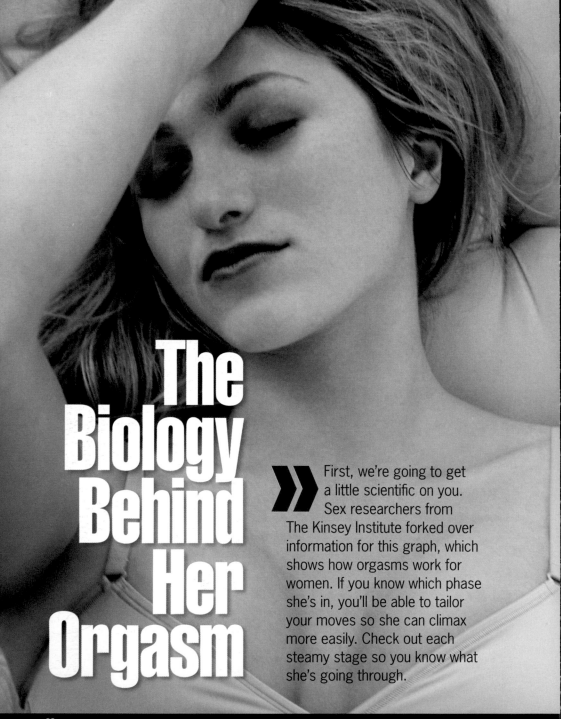

The Biology Behind Her Orgasm

>> First, we're going to get a little scientific on you. Sex researchers from The Kinsey Institute forked over information for this graph, which shows how orgasms work for women. If you know which phase she's in, you'll be able to tailor your moves so she can climax more easily. Check out each steamy stage so you know what she's going through.

Plateau

Once she's aroused, she reaches a bit of a standstill…and if you don't make the right moves, she may never hit that ultimate goal. That's because her body has gotten used to whatever you were doing during the excitement phase and needs different kinds of stimulation to get hot enough to peak. It's important to switch up your moves and not stick with the same pattern of touching, licking, or thrusting.

Orgasm

When she climaxes, it'll often come on suddenly and last for about 15 to 18 seconds. You'll feel her vaginal muscles flexing involuntarily, her feet will likely spasm, and she may develop a flush across her chest.

Resolution

During this phase, the body is slowly returning to its normal state. Feel-good hormones like dopamine and oxytocin are racing through her body, making her feel happy and relaxed.

Excitement

As soon as you start touching her in a sexy way, she gets excited, and her body shows physical signs of it: Her skin becomes flushed, her nipples harden, and she begins to get wet down there.

The Different Kinds of Os

>> Men are sexually simple. We don't mean that as an insult—in fact, we envy you! But you likely have one type of peak, and that's it. Females, on the other hand, are way more complicated. "Women can have various kinds of orgasms, and they all feel different," says sexologist Sadie Allison, author of *Ride 'Em Cowgirl*. "What type she has really depends on where and how she's stimulated." And though you'll never be able to have these Os, it's a good idea to understand each kind so you know how to give them to the woman in your life. Here they are.

CLITORAL

This is the most common type for a woman to have. But don't think that just because it's the usual, it's less special. Trust us, it feels *sooo* good. To give her one, stimulate her clitoris during sex—it's easy to do this in girl-on-top, since her love button will be right in front of you. The key is to start slowly and then rub more a little more aggressively.

G-SPOT

Women often describe this climax as feeling deeper or more intense. To give her one of these, you have to stimulate her G-spot during sex. We've already told you where that is, but here's a reminder: It's situated about 2 inches up on the front wall of her vagina. You can hit this spot with your finger to push her to her limit, or you can try it during sex by using the missionary position. Just prop up her butt with a few pillows so her pelvis is at the right angle to let you hit the area.

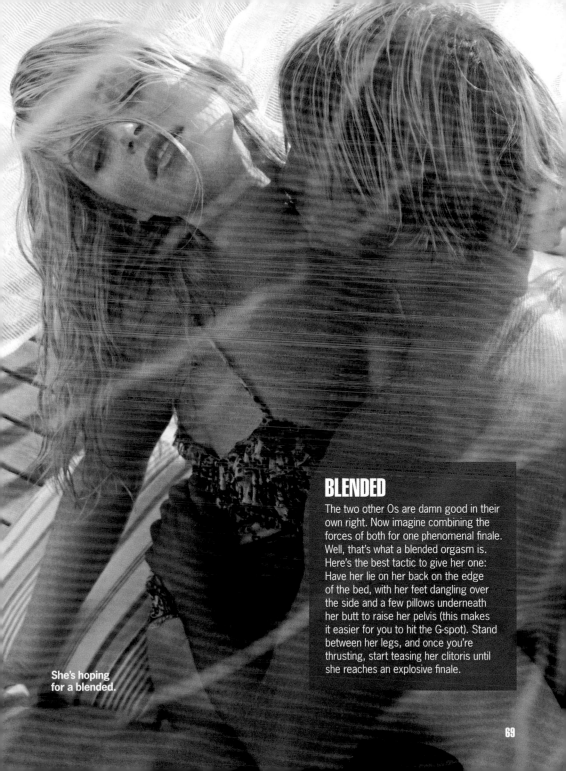

BLENDED

The two other Os are damn good in their own right. Now imagine combining the forces of both for one phenomenal finale. Well, that's what a blended orgasm is. Here's the best tactic to give her one: Have her lie on her back on the edge of the bed, with her feet dangling over the side and a few pillows underneath her butt to raise her pelvis (this makes it easier for you to hit the G-spot). Stand between her legs, and once you're thrusting, start teasing her clitoris until she reaches an explosive finale.

She's hoping
for a blended.

Are You Big or Small?

>> Having an anaconda in your pants is nice, but it doesn't automatically make it more likely that she'll orgasm. And on the flip side, if your penis is a bit smaller, it doesn't mean you won't be able to please her. Here are some tips for those who fall a bit above or below average.

▶ If You're Smaller Than Average

There are actually benefits to having some, er, shortcomings in the size department. "A smaller penis tends to fit nicely against many women's G-spot, whereas larger guys may miss it completely," says Joy Davidson, PhD, author of *Fearless Sex*. Here's the perfect position: Get her in doggie-style, and have her lean down on her elbows so your hips are higher than hers (like the Hang Ten in our Kama Sutra chapter). This will make your package rub right against that pleasure spot. Also, don't forget about your hands. "If you or she rubs her clitoris during sex, it enhances the intercourse and your size becomes a nonissue," says Davidson.

▶ If You're Larger Than Average

As we mentioned earlier, her vagina is built to stretch and accommodate you. So unless you're measuring upward of 12 or 13 inches, having bigger junk won't be a problem. However, lube is a must for a guy like you—it'll make for a smoother entry if she's feeling a bit tight. Also, positions that allow you to go really deep may be uncomfortable for her. Instead, it's a good idea to let her be on top so she can determine how much of you is comfortable to take in. And have sex with her as much as possible (what a drag, right?). "Think of sex as a workout for her vaginal muscles," says Davidson. "The more she does it, the better they become at stretching."

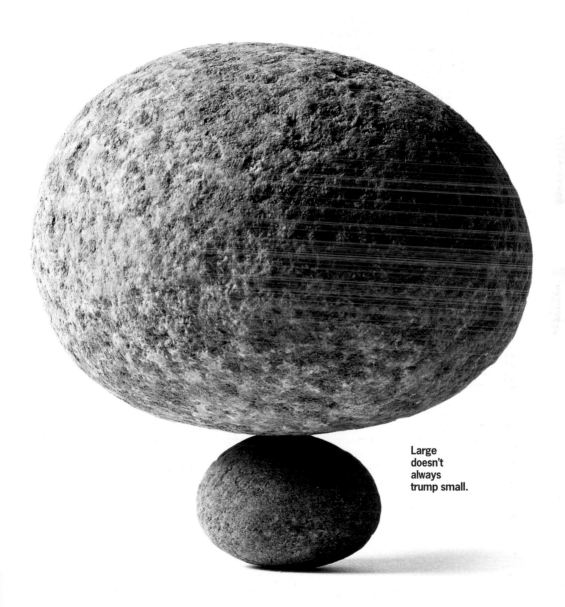

Large
doesn't
always
trump small.

What You Should Know About Thrusting

>> Women love men who can dance. It's not because they want someone they can show off. They figure if you can move your hips on the dance floor, you'll know how to use them in bed. See, ladies need a variety of speeds and rhythms to reach climax. And the better your hip action, the more likely she is to call you the mattress king. Here are some techniques that go beyond the basic in-and-out that you should be aware of.

THE CORKSCREW

Think about how you twist a screw in. Do the same motion with your penis and you'll rock her world. There is a reason they call it screwing, after all. Go as deep as possible inside her, then rotate your hips in a big circle. You'll hit parts of her vaginal walls that straight in-and-out thrusting miss, and your pelvis will grind against her clitoris for double pleasure.

SATISFY A WOMAN—EVERY. SINGLE. TIME.

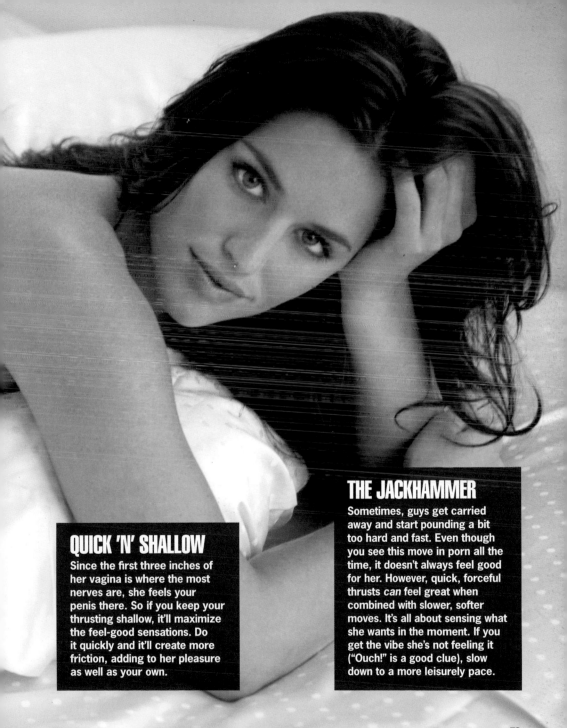

QUICK 'N' SHALLOW

Since the first three inches of her vagina is where the most nerves are, she feels your penis there. So if you keep your thrusting shallow, it'll maximize the feel-good sensations. Do it quickly and it'll create more friction, adding to her pleasure as well as your own.

THE JACKHAMMER

Sometimes, guys get carried away and start pounding a bit too hard and fast. Even though you see this move in porn all the time, it doesn't always feel good for her. However, quick, forceful thrusts *can* feel great when combined with slower, softer moves. It's all about sensing what she wants in the moment. If you get the vibe she's not feeling it ("Ouch!" is a good clue), slow down to a more leisurely pace.

73

Stay in Her While Switching Positions

Want to seem like a smooth lover who's in complete control? Master this move and take her from one position to the next without knocking heads and tangling bodies. Trust us, it will impress her.

1 Start in missionary close to the edge of the left side of the bed.

2 Grab her left leg, and wrap it around your waist.

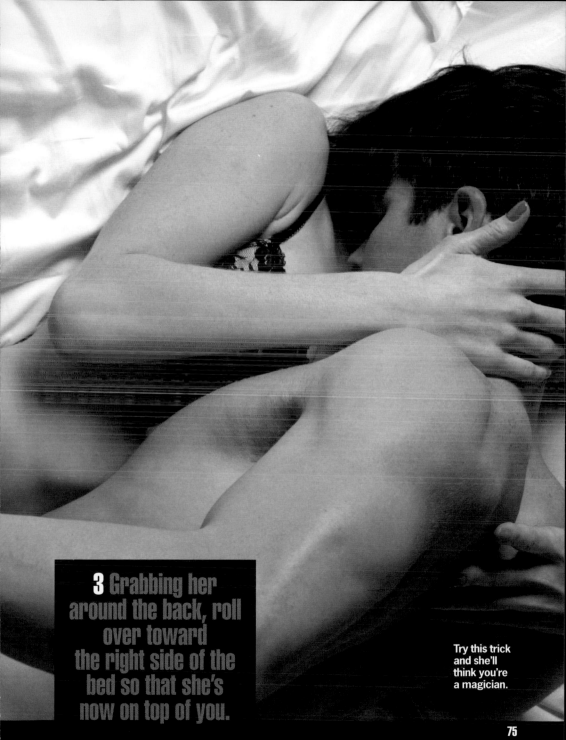

3 Grabbing her around the back, roll over toward the right side of the bed so that she's now on top of you.

Try this trick and she'll think you're a magician.

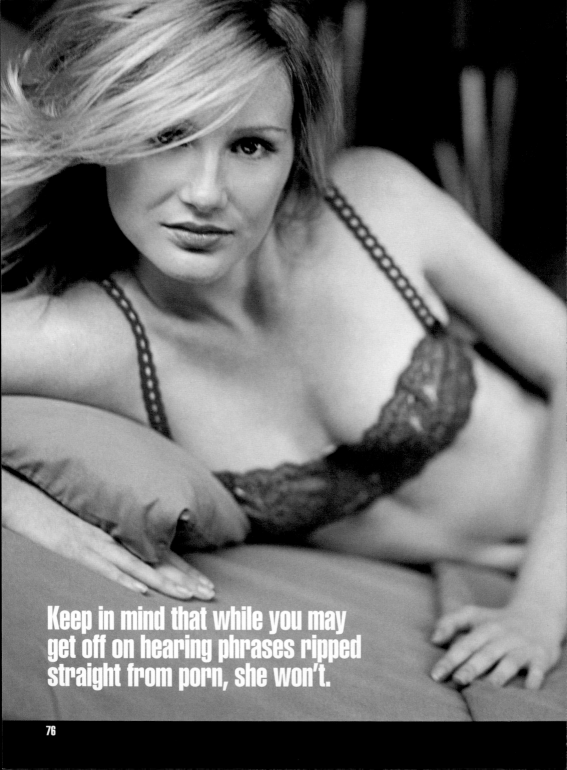

Keep in mind that while you may get off on hearing phrases ripped straight from porn, she won't.

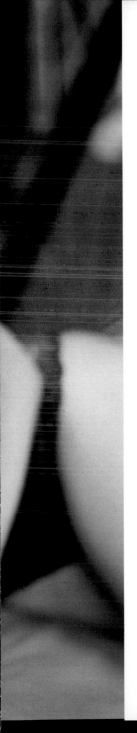

What to Say in Bed

>> "Uttering something naughty to her midact can really heighten the entire experience," says Aline Zoldbrod, PhD, coauthor of Sex Talk. "It makes her feel more desirable, and that contributes to her climaxing more easily." But keep in mind that while you might get off on hearing phrases ripped straight from porn, most chicks prefer things that won't make them feel like a hooker. We asked real women and found out the top things they want to hear you say…and what totally turns them off.

SAY...

"You're *sooo* hot!"

"Do you like it like that?"

"I love going down on you."

"You taste so good."

DON'T SAY...

"Did you come yet?"

"Who's your daddy?"

"Now that I've gone down on you..."

"Time to get waxed"

Try Using a

Maybe take
the dog
off the bed
first....

Vibrator in Bed

>> Men have strong opinions on bringing a vibrator into sex, and we realize this is dicey territory for some. But a recent study shows that a majority of guys are willing to try out a buzzy toy in bed. If you are a little weirded out, it's probably because you're worried it'll replace *you* between the sheets...but it really just enhances everything for her (and you!). These are the best ways to bring a vibe to bed.

During oral, hold the side of the vibrator against your cheek as you lick her clitoris. It'll make your tongue quiver even more and feel unexpected and arousing for her.

While using your mouth to pleasure her, put the vibrator inside her so it's slightly angled toward her belly button—this way, it'll hit her G-spot.

If it's small enough, set it on low and place it between your penis and testicles during sex. The vibrations feel great against your balls, and it'll reverberate through your girl as you move in and out of her.

While she's on top, use it on her clitoris. Start with the slowest speed, and as she gets more excited, turn it up to full blast.

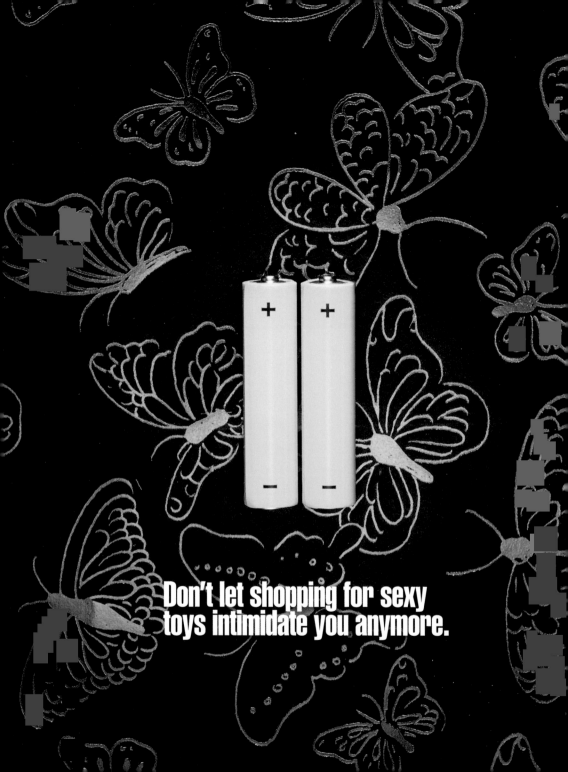

Don't let shopping for sexy
toys intimidate you anymore.

The Best Vibrators to Use as a Couple

Shopping for a toy can be a bit intimidating, especially for a guy. And that's totally understandable—it might feel a bit freaky being in a room full of penis look-alikes. These are the best options for couples, and not a single one resembles (or could compete with) your junk.

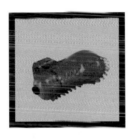

Shag Factory Finger Vibe

Slip the soft plastic over your finger, and use it to rub her clitoris. It is unobtrusive and has three speeds to switch things up.

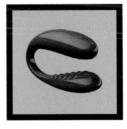

The We-Vibe

This best seller is great because it's totally hands-free. The thinner part goes inside her and presses against her G-spot; the other end goes against her clitoris. The best part? It's small enough that you can penetrate her while it's inside her…and you'll get to feel some of those awesome vibrations too.

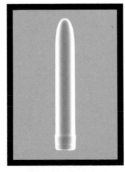

Jimmyjane Iconic Smoothie

This slick tube is ideal for clitoral or vaginal stimulation. And she can use it by running its small tip over your penis.

Have Extra-Intimate Sex

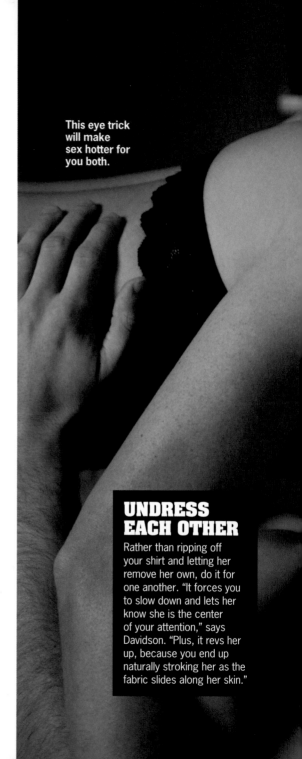

This eye trick will make sex hotter for you both.

>> Wild hookups that leave you both winded and worried that the neighbors heard are a blast. But sometimes, she craves sex that brings you closer and makes you both feel romantic. "If she's giving you signs that that's what she wants, the key is engaging with each other at every stage so you feel like you're a single unit rather than two separate entities," says Joy Davidson, PhD. These little moves will help boost that intimacy while getting it on.

UNDRESS EACH OTHER

Rather than ripping off your shirt and letting her remove her own, do it for one another. "It forces you to slow down and lets her know she is the center of your attention," says Davidson. "Plus, it revs her up, because you end up naturally stroking her as the fabric slides along her skin."

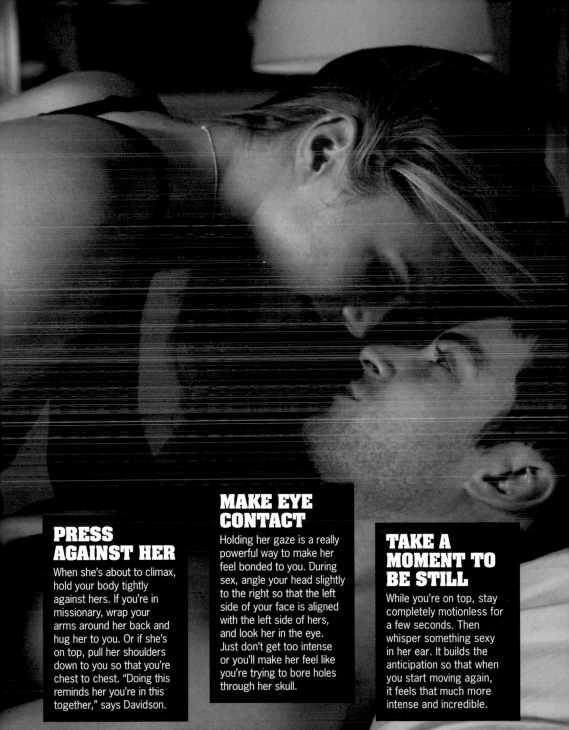

PRESS AGAINST HER

When she's about to climax, hold your body tightly against hers. If you're in missionary, wrap your arms around her back and hug her to you. Or if she's on top, pull her shoulders down to you so that you're chest to chest. "Doing this reminds her you're in this together," says Davidson.

MAKE EYE CONTACT

Holding her gaze is a really powerful way to make her feel bonded to you. During sex, angle your head slightly to the right so that the left side of your face is aligned with the left side of hers, and look her in the eye. Just don't get too intense or you'll make her feel like you're trying to bore holes through her skull.

TAKE A MOMENT TO BE STILL

While you're on top, stay completely motionless for a few seconds. Then whisper something sexy in her ear. It builds the anticipation so that when you start moving again, it feels that much more intense and incredible.

Sync Your Orgasms

» Climaxing at the same time may seem as elusive as winning the lottery, but it's actually not as hard as you think. And the benefit is that it makes you feel even more connected. "Having an orgasm within seconds of each other is one of the most gratifying sexual encounters you can have," says Ian Kerner, PhD. "Every sensation is amplified since you're experiencing it in tandem."

Since men tend to finish faster than women do, it's important to slow down until she catches up. If you feel yourself coming close, take a quick break and make a ring around the tip of your penis using your thumb and pointer finger, and squeeze gently. This will slow blood flow and temporarily dull the sensation you feel, so you don't blow your load too soon. Or you can stop and change positions to let yourself cool down a bit.

Once you notice that she's on the verge, go full force: Thrust harder to create feel-good friction that'll send you both into that blissful state. If she's already spiraling out of control and you want to catch up, watch her face. Seeing how you've brought her to this state will help you get off.

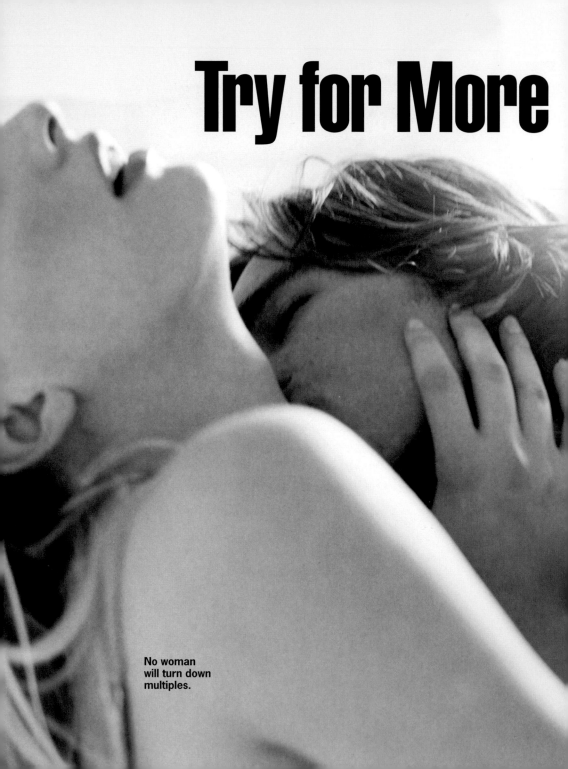

Try for More

No woman
will turn down
multiples.

Than One Climax

Since achieving one orgasm is a pretty big deal for most women, giving her multiples will make you a sex god. Awesome news for you: Once she's reached that first peak, it's actually easier to get her to a second…and third. "The average woman is built to come again and again," says Rachel Carlton Abrams, MD, coauthor of *The Multi-Orgasmic Woman*. "Women don't require the recovery period men do, so they're able to stay aroused for longer, making it easier to reach that additional orgasm." Like anything good, it'll take a little time and effort on your part, but we promise that it will be well worth it. Consider this your road map.

GIVE HER THE FIRST O...

Bring her to orgasm through oral sex. "Making her have one before intercourse means that her body will be geared up to come again," says Abrams. "And because her whole body wakes up after climaxing, she'll respond even more to vaginal stimulation once you penetrate."

...THEN MAKE HER HEAD SPIN WITH ANOTHER ONE...

Give her a few minutes to settle down, but keep her engaged by caressing her breasts. After a few minutes, start having sex. In order to get her to have another orgasm, treat it as a full-contact sport: As you thrust, run your hands over her chest, kiss her neck, or massage her butt. "Women are likelier to have multiples if they're entire body is being stimulated," explains Abrams.

...AND FINISH OFF WITH A THIRD

After giving her another mini break, bring her to the finish line one more time by using your hands. "By this point, her body will be hypersensitive, so you'll have to take care," says Abrams. "Your fingers are the best instruments to do that because you can really control how much pressure you use." Start extremely softly, lightly moving them over her clitoris. As she gets into it, use a firmer touch until she explodes.

THE DIRTY DOZEN: Positions for Her Pleasure

>> We rounded up the different passion poses every man should have in his repertoire. These hit all the right spots for her (and you!) and will sure as hell help her orgasm.

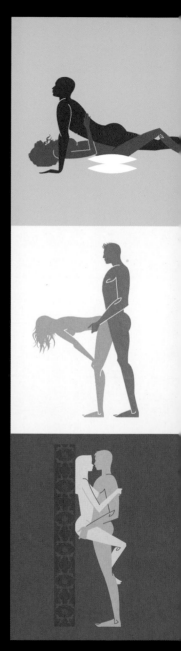

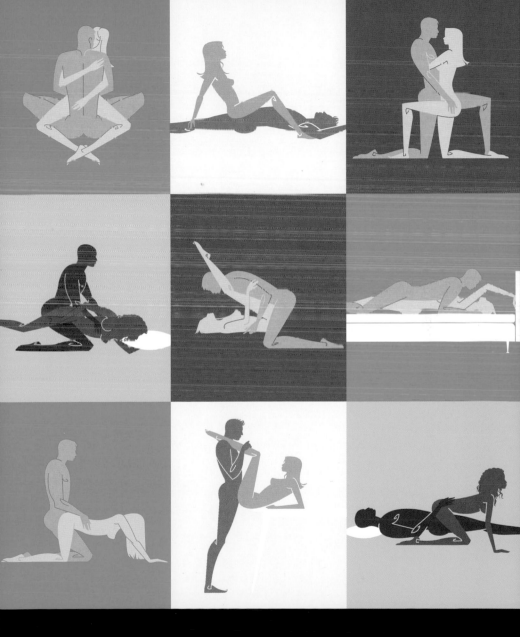

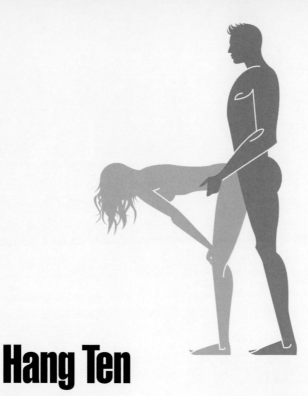

Hang Ten

How to Do It
Stand up, and have her stand in front of you. Ask her to bend over at the waist, with her legs spread slightly, her back straight, and her hands resting on her knees for support. Enter her from behind, and hold her hips for leverage.

Why She'll Love It
Your hands are free to stimulate her breasts. Plus, unlike in other from-behind positions, your legs and torsos touch, making her feel close to you.

Why It's Good for You
Her being bent forward lets you go extra deep.

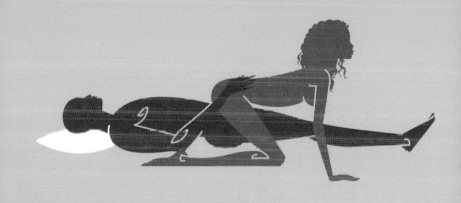

Back-Up Boogie

How to Do It

Lie on your back, with your legs straight in front of you and a pillow under your head. Have her straddle you, with her head facing your feet. She should put her hands on the floor for support as she backs up onto your penis. Hold her upper thighs while she thrusts up and down the entire length of your shaft.

Why She'll Love It

It's a mix of doggie-style and girl-on-top. The combo lets her control the speed and depth and lets you hit her G-spot.

Why It's Good for You

Since your head is elevated by the pillow, you get a fantastic view of her ass moving up and down.

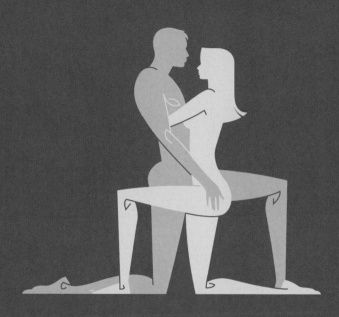

Passion Pretzel

How to Do It

Start by kneeling face-to-face with each other. Each of you should place the opposite foot flat on the ground and nudge closer, joining genitals. Then, leaning forward on your planted foot, both of you lunge back and forth for a slow, upright romp.

Why She'll Love It

The leisurely torso-to-torso grind provides great clitoral stimulation.

Why It's Good for You

You're in the exact same position, so you get to share the workload evenly—meaning you can really focus on your own pleasure while knowing she's having fun.

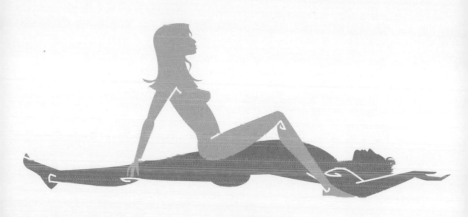

Joystick Joyride

How to Do It
Lie on your back, with her on top. Tell her to lean back so her elbows rest on either side of your knees. As she moves back and forth with your penis inside her, you'll have prime access to rub her clitoris.

Why She'll Love It
By having her lean back, your penis rubs against her G-spot. And like we said, you can stimulate her clitoris, almost guaranteeing an orgasm.

Why It's Good for You
Her leaned-back pose will give you an amazingly graphic view.

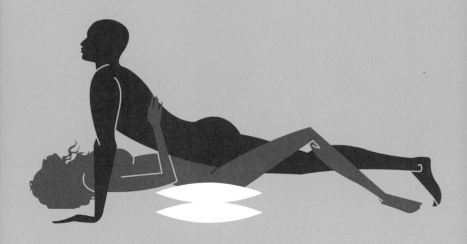

Figure Eight

How to Do It

Have her lie on her back, with a pillow under her butt and her knees bent and open. Plant your hands on either side of her head, and enter her. Instead of thrusting, gyrate your hips in a figure-eight motion (it allows her to feel your whole package).

Why She'll Love It

Her elevated pelvis means your pubic bone will gently rub against her clitoris.

Why It's Good for You

The circular motion feels unique and surprising. And according to experts, new sensations up the erotic factor.

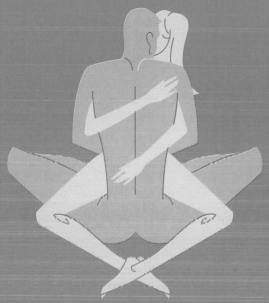

Get Down on It

How to Do It
Sit cross-legged on the floor or your bed. Have her sit in your lap so she's facing you, with her legs wrapped around your back. Then both of you should rock back and forth.

Why She'll Love It
Her entire body is pressed against yours, so all of it is being aroused. And you can have a long make-out session during sex since you're face-to-face.

Why It's Good for You
Being so close means your penis is able to go as deep as possible.

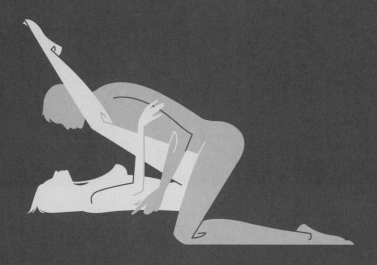

Rock 'n' Roll

How to Do It

Have her lie faceup and bring her knees up to her chin. Lie on top of her so she can rest her legs against your shoulders as you thrust in and out of her.

Why She'll Love It

This alternate man-on-top position makes her feel open and vulnerable, and your deep thrusts will feel amazing for her.

Why It's Good for You

There's nothing standing between you and her vagina—you have free rein to thrust and go as deep or shallow as you want.

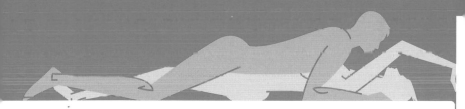

Reach for the Heavens

How to Do It

Ask her to lie on her back with her arms over her head, grasping the top of the mattress or your headboard. Enter her missionary-style, and then have her bring her legs together tightly. With her thighs closed, your penis will rub against her labia and clitoris every time you move.

Why She'll Love It

This feels so good because it allows you to do what experts call the Coital Alignment Technique (CAT). What's that? It's any position that allows the base of your penis or pubic bone to make consistent contact with her clitoris. And being in missionary with her legs tightly closed does exactly this. Keep up a steady thrusting rhythm and you'll definitely blow her mind. The best part: A study showed that when the CAT is used, women experience a 56 percent increase in orgasms. Plus, with her legs closed, it'll create lots of feel-good friction for you.

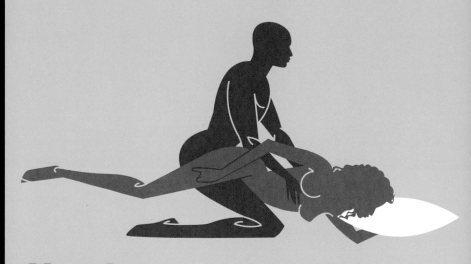

Linguine

How to Do It

Have her lie on her side, putting a pillow under her head for support. Kneel directly behind her butt, leaning slightly over her body. Push one of your knees between her legs, positioning your body so you can penetrate.

Why She'll Love It

You'll easily hit her G-spot, and the half-spooning position feels very intimate.

Why It's Good for You

Her hands are totally free to roam behind her and gently play with your testicles.

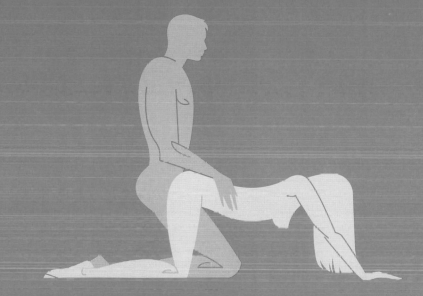

G-Spot Jiggy

How to Do It
Have her get down on all fours, with you behind her and plunging into her. You can grab her butt to help control your thrusting.

Why She'll Love It
The downward angle grants you easy access to her G-spot. Also, she's free to reach down and play with her clitoris as you pump away.

Why It's Good for You
The downward angle creates tons of friction against your shaft.

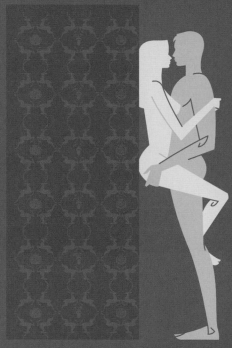

Stand and Deliver

How to Do It

She should stand against a wall with her legs spread slightly. Face her, grab the backs of her thighs (where her butt meets her legs), and lift her so she can wrap her legs around your waist. She can push her back against the wall for leverage as you thrust.

Why She'll Love It

Your woman will feel hotter than ever in this pose because it has a take-me-now quality to it.

Why It's Good for You

Between lifting her up and pushing her against a wall, you will feel like the ultimate man doing this one.

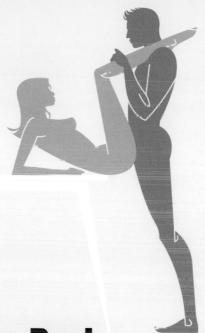

Sneak-a-Peek

How to Do It
Have her lie down on the kitchen table so her butt is right at the edge. Stand in front of her to enter her, and bring her legs up and over your shoulders. You can grab her hips or booty to help you thrust.

Why She'll Love It
Putting her legs over your shoulders gives her leverage, so she can slow you down or speed you up if she wants.

Why It's Good for You
Her pelvis naturally tilts in this pose, allowing you to sink into her deeper.

CHAPTER 5

UH-OH, SOMETHING WENT WRONG

When you're close to coming, pretty much nothing can stop you. Your Great Aunt Gerty could walk in wearing a bustier and you'd probably still finish. But women? Lots can derail them. Here's what to do if it goes awry.

»

She's Lost Her Orgasm
(Get It Back, Stat!)

》》 As we mentioned earlier, a woman can be *thisclose* to climaxing and then—poof!— it's gone. Don't take offense; it's just one of those things that happens every now and then, and it may have nothing to do with you. One common reason is that she loses her focus. Another is that a change of pace just isn't working for her. Rest assured, it's a fixable problem…and you *can* get her back on track.

TRY RESETTING

If she was really close and then you changed positions or rhythm, stopping and restarting can get her back in the zone. "Pull out, and just kiss her," says sex therapist Gloria Brame, PhD. "After a while, you can start up again." In the future, to make sure you don't switch it up when she's on the brink, whisper "Tell me when you're close" at some point midsex. That'll encourage her to be more vocal and let you know when a move is working for her.

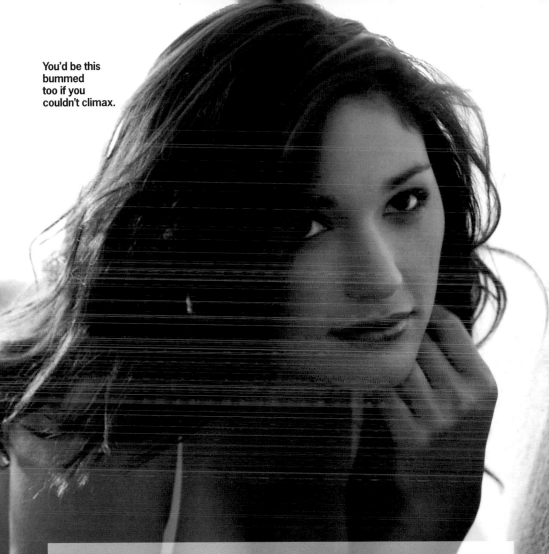

You'd be this bummed too if you couldn't climax.

CLEAR HER MIND

Women are way more prone to getting distracted by little things during sex than men are. She may be thinking, *Do I look fat at this angle?* or *Is he having fun?* or even *Did I remember to lock the front door?* Those thoughts can completely knock her off course because they take her out of the moment. Take some preventative measures by making sure wherever you are having sex is as serene as possible. "Turn off your cell phone, put on music, and dim the lights to make her feel less self-conscious and help her stay in the moment," says Brame. "And if you sense her starting to lose focus, engage her. Give her a deep kiss to bring her back to the task at hand or start talking to her about what you're going to do next." This will force her to stay connected, and her mind won't wander.

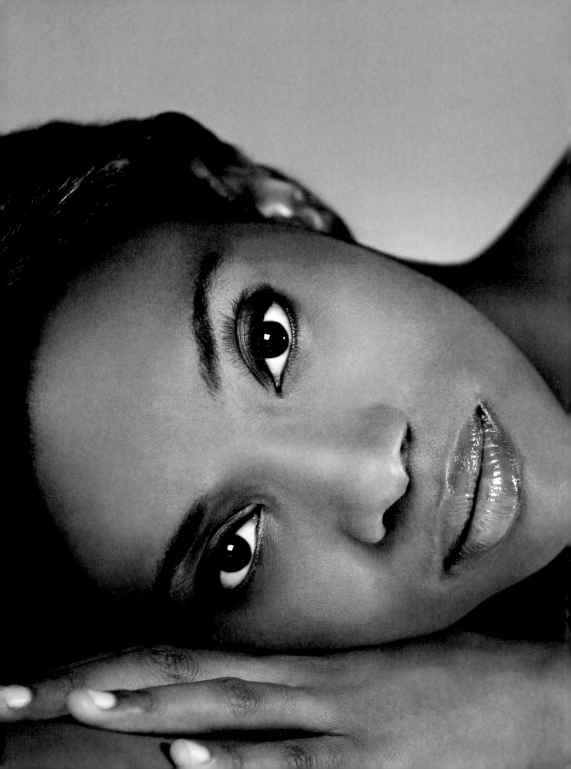

Talk About Sex

» You're probably thinking that the only kind of sexy convo you want to participate in is the dirty variety. We get it—dissecting what went on between the sheets can be awkward. However, if you want to suss out what it takes to make her come, sometimes the only way to do it is by having a chat (of course, we tell women to do the same in almost every issue of Cosmo!). Here are a few ideas for having those talks in the heat of the moment and right after.

During the Deed

- To see if she likes your technique, pause and ask "Want that again?" If she says yes, she's into it...but if she hesitates, she's not loving it.

- Give her options. Ask "Is it better like this or that?" Both answers will be positive, so she won't feel bad picking a fave.

- Say "It feels so good when you..." Hearing you open up will make her feel okay reciprocating.

- Have playful sex. It's a lot easier to talk midsession when the mood is light than when the intensity is sky-high.

Post Pleasure

- In that afterglow period, kiss her neck and tell her what you enjoyed most. The touch makes you both feel more connected, and since you went first, she'll feel okay opening up.

- Be totally honest and say "I want to make you feel even better next time. What can I do?" She'll appreciate how truthful you're being and love that your goal is to make her happy in bed.

- Pick one specific point of her technique, and ask her to rate from 1 to 10 how warm/cold she thinks it would feel. She'll be more at ease having the conversation that way and be honest.

Sometimes, It Just Won't Happen

Occasionally, no matter what you do, she won't be able to climax. "A variety of factors could be at play when this happens," says Ian Kerner, PhD. "It might be that she's stressed or on a medication that's throwing her body out of whack. And sometimes, it just won't happen no matter how much she likes what you're doing." So many things have to align for a woman to orgasm that every once in a while, one slips through the cracks. "The best thing to do is not let it eat at your psyche," says Kerner. You could even ask her if anything is wrong—a woman will be flattered if she feels like you are that concerned that she didn't have fun. Also, by bringing it up, you open the doors of communication, so she can tell you if it was something you did that made her unable to finish or if it was just a random thing, explains Kerner.

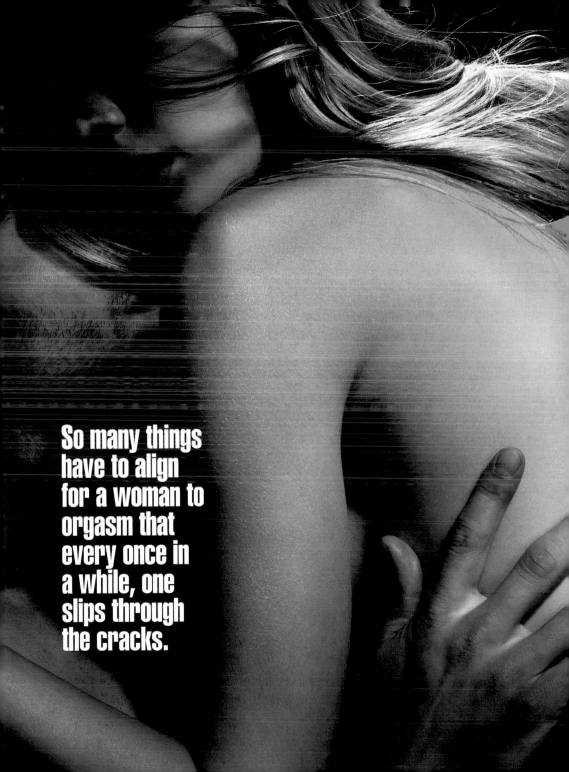

So many things have to align for a woman to orgasm that every once in a while, one slips through the cracks.

Fix Your Sex Flub

>> We've all been there: The mood is hot, things are going well in bed, and suddenly, something embarrassing or weird happens and kills the mood. Have no fear: We found solutions to the most common bed bloopers.

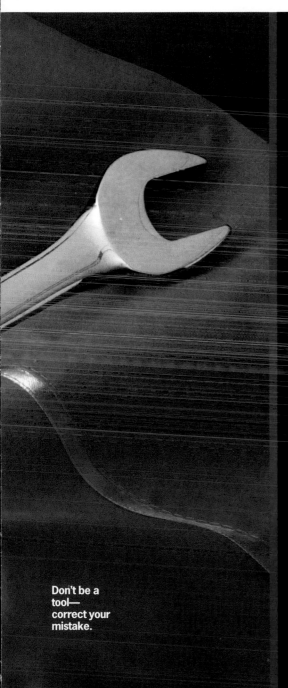

Don't be a tool—correct your mistake.

You Used Way Too Much Lube

So you went a little squeeze-happy with the lubricant bottle, and now her V zone is more like a Slip 'n Slide. Instead of trying to wipe it off, suggest getting down in the shower. The water will add a fun dynamic and wash away the extra stuff you squirted on.

You Went for the Wrong Hole

We understand: Sometimes in the heat of passion, you accidentally try to enter the wrong spot (they *are* close together, after all!). Don't stress. Just wash up really fast to avoid spreading bacteria, and go for the right place the next time. Nothing's worse than a guy who continually pokes at your back door, thinking it's your vagina.

You Let a Fart Slip

There are two options here. One, pretend it didn't happen, and ignore it. She'll be happy to follow your lead if it doesn't reek enough for her to need a gas mask. Or you can crack a joke about it to make her giggle and relax even more. However, if she queefs, ignore it—laughing about *that* will make her feel uncomfortable.

You Take Too Long With the Condom

It's a bit of a bummer to be in the heat of things and then have to wait while a guy fishes around for a condom, has trouble opening the wrapper, and then takes forever to put it on. First, always have condoms by your bedside, so you can grab them quickly. And if you fumble while putting it on, don't worry. We'd rather you do it right! You can keep things simmering by saying something like "I can't wait to get inside you."

You Finished...but She Didn't

You tried to last, but something came over you and you ejaculated before she came. It's not a big deal...as long as you help her finish. Switch tactics by going down on her or pulling out her vibrator until she has an orgasm.

Moves That Freak Her Out

>> It's not easy for her to tell you if some of your skills leave something to be desired. She doesn't want to hurt your feelings, and she might be afraid you'll get mad. But since you want to become a mattress rock star, you should know this stuff. Here are the two biggest that could keep her from finishing.

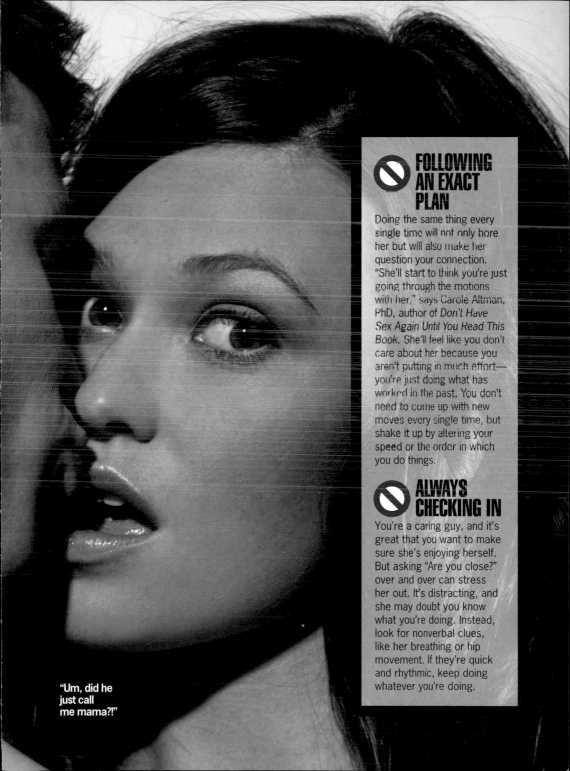

FOLLOWING AN EXACT PLAN

Doing the same thing every single time will not only bore her but will also make her question your connection. "She'll start to think you're just going through the motions with her," says Carole Altman, PhD, author of *Don't Have Sex Again Until You Read This Book*. She'll feel like you don't care about her because you aren't putting in much effort— you're just doing what has worked in the past. You don't need to come up with new moves every single time, but shake it up by altering your speed or the order in which you do things.

ALWAYS CHECKING IN

You're a caring guy, and it's great that you want to make sure she's enjoying herself. But asking "Are you close?" over and over can stress her out. It's distracting, and she may doubt you know what you're doing. Instead, look for nonverbal clues, like her breathing or hip movement. If they're quick and rhythmic, keep doing whatever you're doing.

"Um, did he just call me mama?!"

Was She Really Satisfied?

>> Women have been known to fake it occasionally. Cosmo has told them not to—it's better if you know what doesn't work! But many chicks worry they'll hurt your feelings, so they continue with the phony act. Curious if she's *really* coming? There are actually physical signs that can clue you in.

Her vaginal walls contract lightly for a few seconds.

Her breath becomes spastic and short in the last few moments of sex.

She has a rosy flush all over her chest.

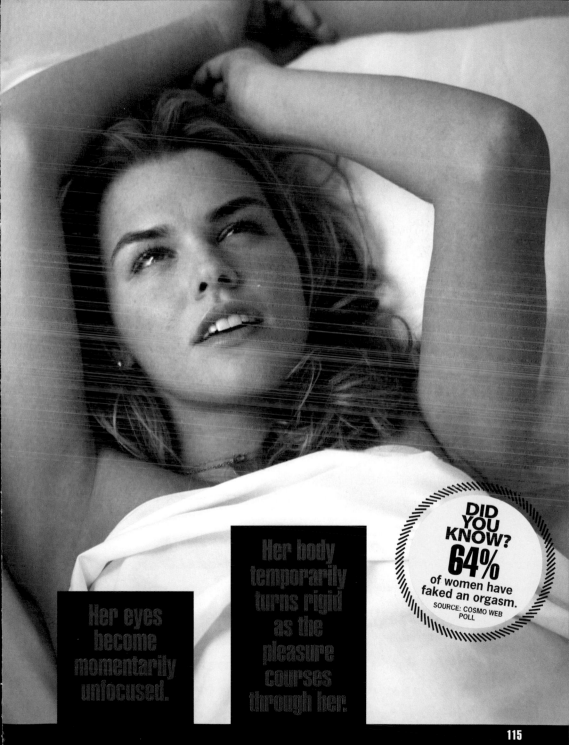

Her eyes become momentarily unfocused.

Her body temporarily turns rigid as the pleasure courses through her.

DID YOU KNOW?
64% of women have faked an orgasm.
SOURCE: COSMO WEB POLL

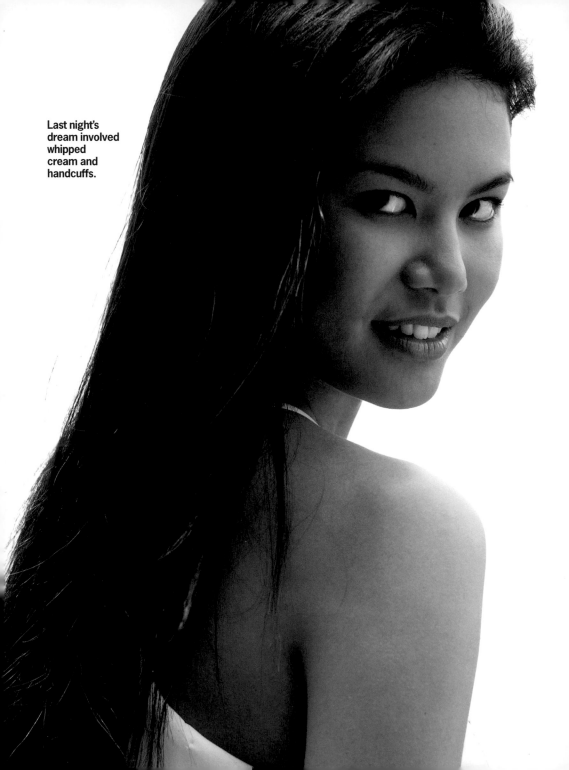

Last night's dream involved whipped cream and handcuffs.

Female Sex Myths, Debunked

>> There are some female sex stereotypes and myths out there that we just *have* to clear up for you. Let some real women explain.

Women Always Want to Cuddle After Sex

"When I'm tired from work, I want to get it on without all the touchy feely stuff."
—Danica, 23

"Sometimes, my body goes into sensory overload after climaxing and I don't want to be touched." —Cassie, 29

They Want You to Initiate It Every Time

"I like being the aggressor. It makes me feel like I'm super powerful if I am the one calling the shots."
—Nina, 22

"I love the look of surprise on his face when we are lying in bed and my hand starts to travel south."
—Tess, 28

Men Crave Sex More Than Women Do

"I want sex just as often as my fiance does. It just tends to be at different times." —Sara, 31

"I like to get it on almost every day. It is a great mood booster and keeps me stress-free." —Monica, 25

Chicks Compare You to Past Flames

"Not true at all. I'm too busy enjoying the guy I am with to think about the last man." —Tara, 24

"If the guy I'm with is having trouble making me orgasm, I think about what he could do better next time, not about what my ex did differently."
—Jessie, 23

Women Don't Have X-Rated Dreams

"Are you kidding?! I have a recurring dream that involves Channing Tatum, handcuffs, and hot wax."
—Ann, 27

"My dreams may not end with a wet spot, but I assure you, some of my best orgasms have happened while I was snoozing." —Deanna, 24

They Want a Guy Who Can Last All Night

"If sex goes on for too long, chafing occurs. I don't want a two-pump chump, but there is such a thing as too long." —Fiona, 32

"I'm happy with 15 to 20 minutes. It's not too short, but it doesn't drag either."
—Stephanie, 27

This lone wolf hasn't had sex in a month!

When You Want It More Than She Does

>> If she doesn't seem as interested in sex as usual, don't take it personally. There are many reasons a woman may not be in the mood as often as you are…and none of them have to do with her not being into you.

You've Been Together for a While

When you're dating someone new, you're practically animals, ready to rip each other's clothes off at any given moment. This is partly because in the early stages, you don't see one another regularly, so you think you have to get it on when you are together. But once you have a steady pattern of hanging out, she may not feel the need to always go at it. She knows you'll be around later, so she isn't as frantic about getting you naked right then.

Feeding into this is the fact that men can get a bit lazy. In the beginning, you feel like you really have to woo her to get her in the sack. But once she's a sure thing, you stop doing some of that stuff (like kissing her out of nowhere or stopping your favorite show because you simply can't be near her without jumping her). Try initiating more spontaneous sex and she'll start feeling that thrill from when you first met. After ordering takeout, pin her to the couch and say you want to see if you can get her off before the food arrives. Or surprise her while she's doing something routine, like ogling her when she's getting dressed on Saturday morning and telling her how unbelievably hot she is. These types of little moves often fall by the wayside as you get more serious. If you start doing them again, it'll get her in the mood.

She's Totally Stressed Out

When she has a lot on her plate at work or is dealing with serious family issues, her first thought won't be hitting the sack with you. If you sense that something is eating at her, it's not the time to push for action. Instead, try to ease the pressure by being affectionate or giving her a massage. It may stop there, but showing her that you care and being understanding just may arouse her.

Her Sex Drive Is Simply Lower Than Yours

Libido is biological to some degree, and it just may be that hers isn't quite as high as yours is. The good news is that a person's sex drive does ebb and flow over the course of a lifetime, so if they aren't equal now, live with it for a bit and hers might match up eventually.

Medical conditions and prescriptions can also cause a drop in sex drive. Being depressed, the type of birth-control pill she's on, and even antibiotics can decrease libido. So it's never a bad idea to encourage her to have a physical and talk to her doctor to make sure everything is okay.

CHAPTER 6

ALL THE KINKY EXTRAS

Now that you have the basics down,
step it up with some of our naughty add-ons.
From bringing in toys to watching porn
together to whipping out the cuffs, we've
got her every erotic fantasy covered.

Other Feel-Good Sensations She'll Love

>> These little moves will literally send shivers racing throughout her body. How can she not think you're the best after that?!

> Swish peppermint schnapps or mouthwash around in your mouth, spit it out, then suck on her nipples. "Both contain alcohol, which adds a tingle. It evaporates quickly, leaving behind an invigorating, skin-tensing sensation," says Carol Queen, PhD, staff sexologist at goodvibes.com.

> Run your fingertips lightly along her inner thighs and the backs of her knees—that skin is sensitive, so even the lightest touch creates a tingling effect.

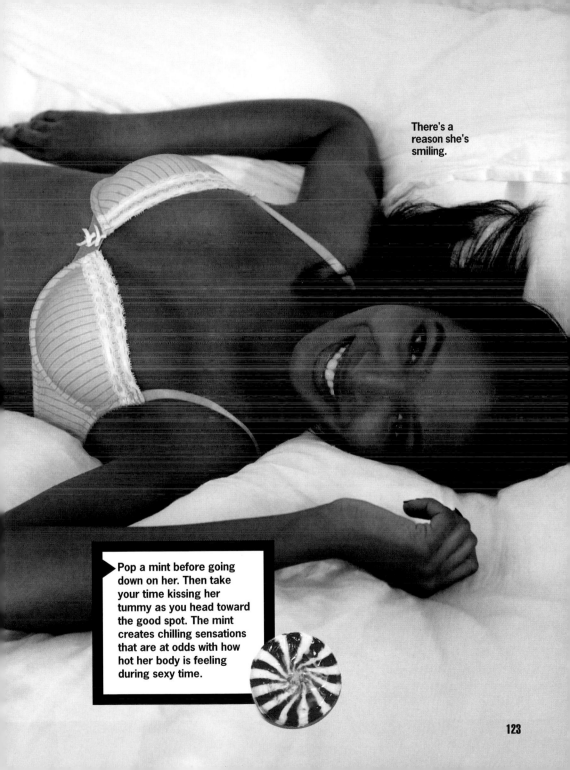

There's a reason she's smiling.

Pop a mint before going down on her. Then take your time kissing her tummy as you head toward the good spot. The mint creates chilling sensations that are at odds with how hot her body is feeling during sexy time.

123

Cuff or Blindfold Her

>> A huge Cosmo poll revealed that more than 60 percent of women have never been handcuffed or blindfolded in bed but would really like to be. And the same percentage of women want to try it on their man yet haven't. You're probably wondering, *If she wants to do it so badly, why she hasn't said anything?* "Many fearless women want to try these fun props but are afraid that you will judge them," says Ian Kerner, PhD. "And even if they're completely at ease with you, they have no idea how to broach the subject." So if you take the lead, she'll not only be grateful... she'll be super excited.

Why It's Hot

First, it's important for you to understand why these kinds of kinky things turn her on. And it's not about being your sex slave. "It allows a woman to completely submit to pleasure," says Carole Altman, PhD. "When she can't move too much or see what's coming, it forces her to think about only the sensations she's experiencing. It also forces her to lie back and enjoy."

And she wants to cuff or blindfold you for the exact opposite reason. "In doing so, she gets to control your pleasure, and it makes her feel really powerful," explains sexologist Sadie Allison.

How to Bring It Up

It's not exactly comfortable to say "So, want me to tie you up later?" in between bites of dinner. Instead, find a lighthearted way to introduce it into sex play. Leave a brightly colored pair of furry handcuffs or a silky scarf on the bed and see what she says. Both are obviously playful and signal that you're looking to have fun. When she catches sight of them, she'll most likely ask about them, and that will open the door for you both to have a conversation about testing them out.

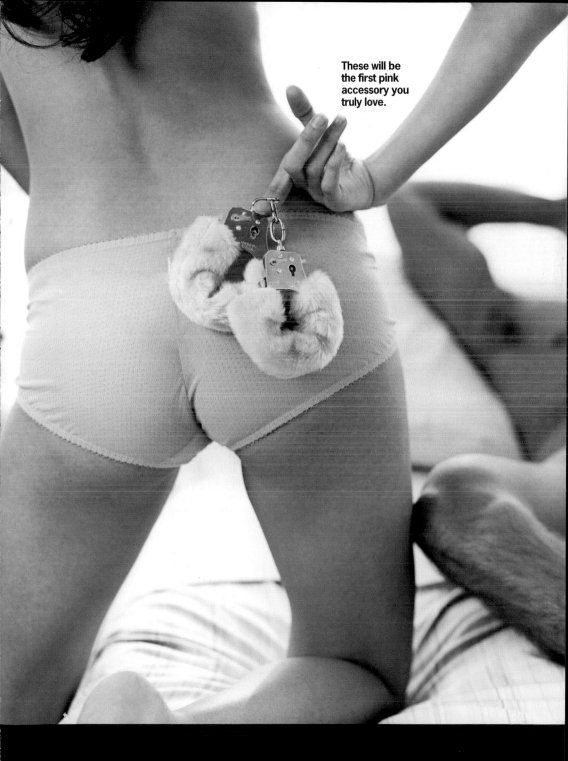

These will be
the first pink
accessory you
truly love.

Her Top Naughty Fantasies

>> Every woman has deep desires that she hasn't necessarily revealed to you. Gentlemen, let us clue you in to some of her top lusty longings.

To Give Up Control

It's a turn-on when a man can show who's boss in bed. Women often feel stressed and like they have a lot of responsibility, so it's arousing to give up control every once in a while. Plus, when you're in the driver's seat, she's better able to lie back and indulge in every sensation.

To Go Buck Wild

Women want to go all out when they're with you; they just worry that a guy will think they're slutty if they get too vocal, reveal their naughtiest fantasy, or introduce a new game. Of course, we know you're an enlightened man who wouldn't think that. But you need to let her know. Tell her how hot it would be if she shared her secret daydream or made wake-the-neighbors noises in bed. Once you do, she'll instantly feel more comfortable letting loose.

To Have a Take-Me-Now Moment

Most of the time, she's going to need a warm-up before diving into the main event. But every now and then, instant gratification is what she craves. That's because spontaneous sex is all that more exhilarating. Also, the fact that you can't wait another second makes her feel totally irresistible.

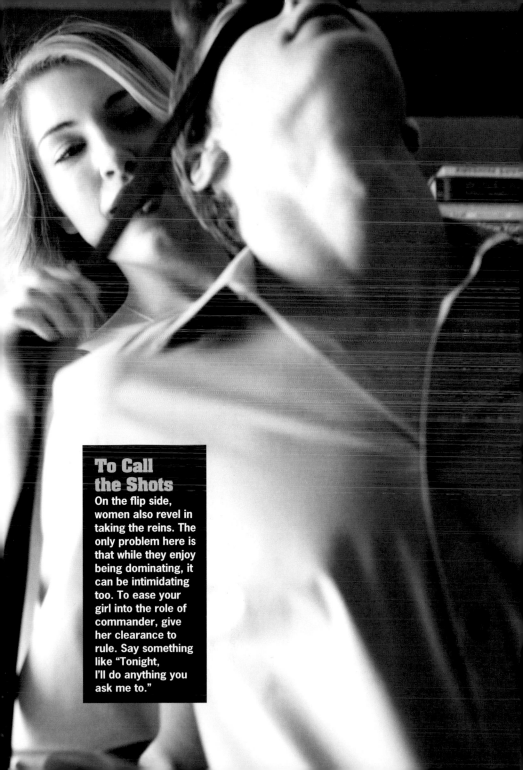

To Call the Shots

On the flip side, women also revel in taking the reins. The only problem here is that while they enjoy being dominating, it can be intimidating too. To ease your girl into the role of commander, give her clearance to rule. Say something like "Tonight, I'll do anything you ask me to."

Go Ahead, Pop In a Porno

》》 Most guys are under the impression that women hate porn. Well, we may not love all the stuff you gravitate toward—like money shots, group sex, and weird fetishes that make you laugh as much as they turn you on—but if you go about it the right way, watching a steamy flick together can be incredibly arousing.

Talk About It

Chat about porn with her to make sure she's comfortable with it. Ask her if she's ever watched it and what her reaction was. If she appears open or curious, go ahead and see if she'd want to watch it with you. And if she seems freaked out by it, let her know that it's something you'd like to do with her but that you want her to feel okay with it, so she should take some time to think about it.

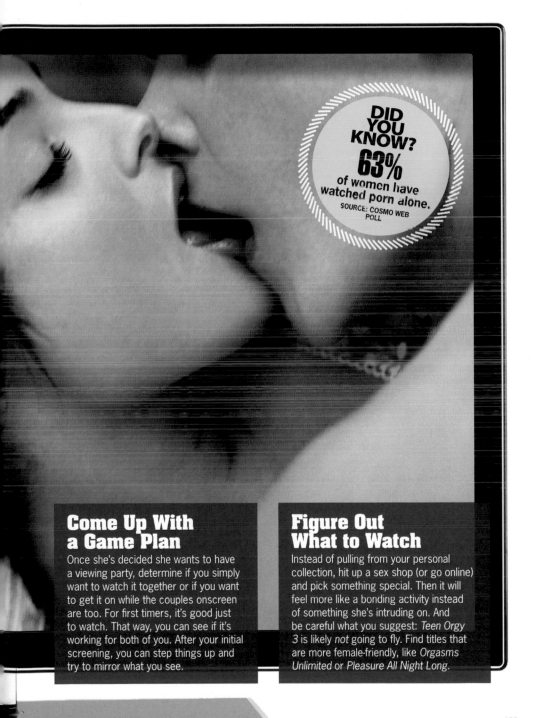

Come Up With a Game Plan

Once she's decided she wants to have a viewing party, determine if you simply want to watch it together or if you want to get it on while the couples onscreen are too. For first timers, it's good just to watch. That way, you can see if it's working for both of you. After your initial screening, you can step things up and try to mirror what you see.

Figure Out What to Watch

Instead of pulling from your personal collection, hit up a sex shop (or go online) and pick something special. Then it will feel more like a bonding activity instead of something she's intruding on. And be careful what you suggest: *Teen Orgy 3* is likely *not* going to fly. Find titles that are more female-friendly, like *Orgasms Unlimited* or *Pleasure All Night Long*.

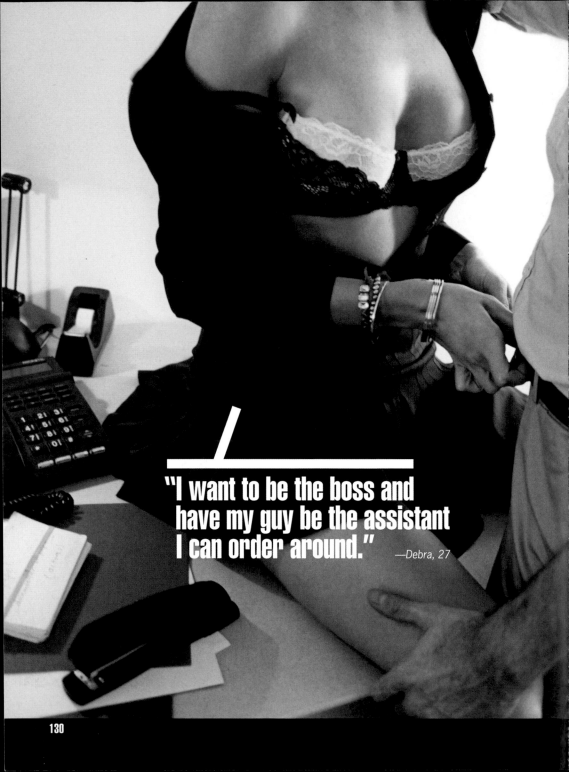

"I want to be the boss and have my guy be the assistant I can order around." —Debra, 27

Role-Playing She's Into

>> Real women share the kinds of roles they're totally into trying out after hours.

"It's cliché, but I love the idea of him being the doctor with me as the nurse." —Kia, 22

"Let's pretend we are two chefs getting extra creative in the kitchen once the restaurant closes for the night." —Candace, 31

"Most guys may find this surprising, but I want to be a stripper and have my man be a customer. There's something very voyeuristic about it. Plus, I'd never strip in real life, so it'd fun to see what it might feel like." —Allison, 26

"I have always thought that photographers are sexy. So I want the guy to pretend to shoot me—the model. The sexier the directions he gives me, the better." —LeAnne, 24

Make Bath Time Sexy

>> Warm water, slippery wet bodies, a steamy room…getting it on in the tub or shower is downright hot. Of course, the confined space and the fact that water washes away her natural lubricants can make things a bit tricky. Luckily for you, certain moves will keep everything going smoothly, making you look like the sex star you are.

Give Her a Sensual Sponge Bath

Begin by peeling off her clothes. Then slide into the tub first, and have her sit between your legs and lie back on your chest. Lather up a loofah or soft sponge with body wash, and slowly trace circles around her breasts then down her tummy and back. Move the sponge lower, and very softly rub it in circular motions between her legs.

Let the Showerhead Do Some Work

Drain the water, and have her lie similarly to how you were before on the tub floor. Let the spray tantalize your bodies. Try pointing the stream so it goes directly between her legs, then play with the water settings to see what she likes best. Just avoid directly spraying her clitoris (it may be too much pressure for that spot). To help her orgasm, kneel by her side and play with her breasts.

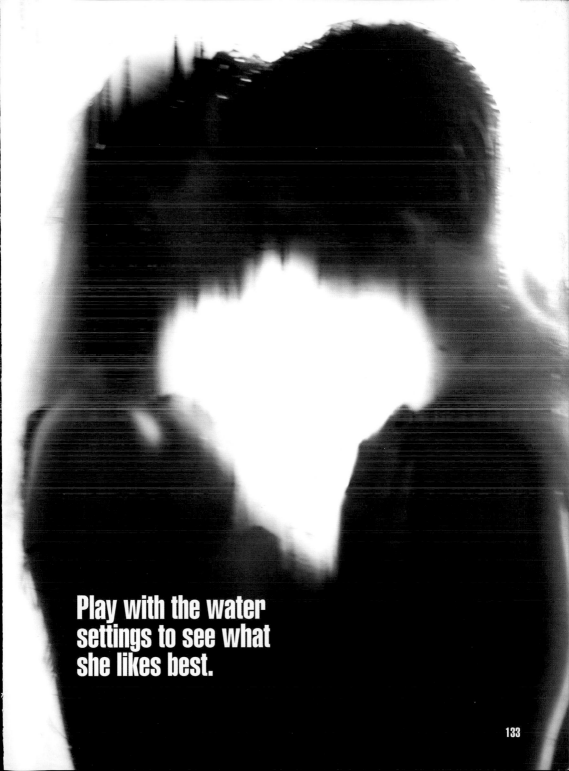

Play with the water
settings to see what
she likes best.

Other Sizzling Toys

>> Vibrators aren't the only gadgets that can boost her arousal. Here are three other sexy accessories to consider.

A MASSAGE CANDLE

As these burn, the wax actually turns into warm massage oil. Drizzle a little onto her back, and give her a rubdown before things really get going.

CHOCOLATE BODY PAINT

This combines two of women's favorite things: chocolate and sex. Brush some onto her breasts, and then slowly lick it off. It's novel, which will make the entire experience seem fun and erotic.

VIBRATING RING

It's a ring that fits around your penis and buzzes. It's small and, therefore, a little less intrusive than a regular vibrator. But it has the same payoff: Her clitoris gets stimulated, and the vibrations feel great against your shaft too.

A FULL-LENGTH MIRROR

You don't even need to hit a sex store for this. Get a mirror that you can put beside the bed every once in a while. Studies suggest that when women are able to watch themselves having sex, they get more aroused than usual.

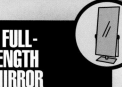

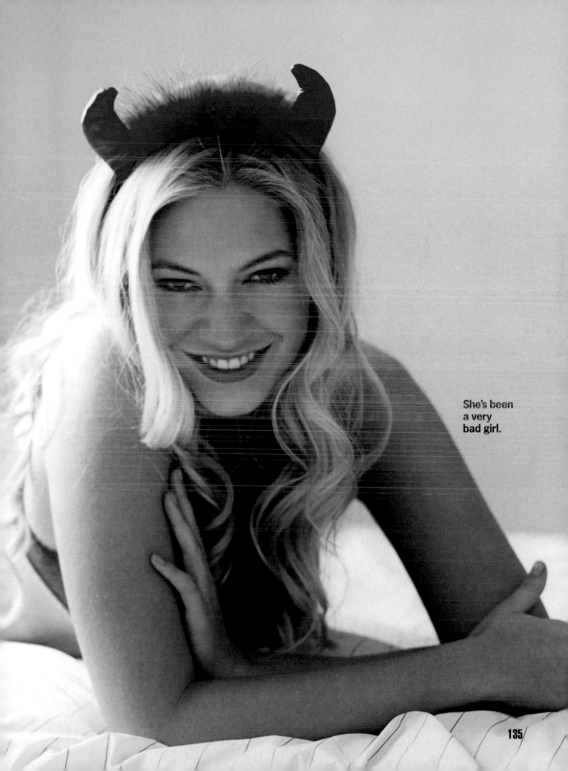

She's been
a very
bad girl.

SEX Q&A

In case we missed
a specific piece of
information you were
looking for in these
pages, we address some
other important questions
we've received from guys.

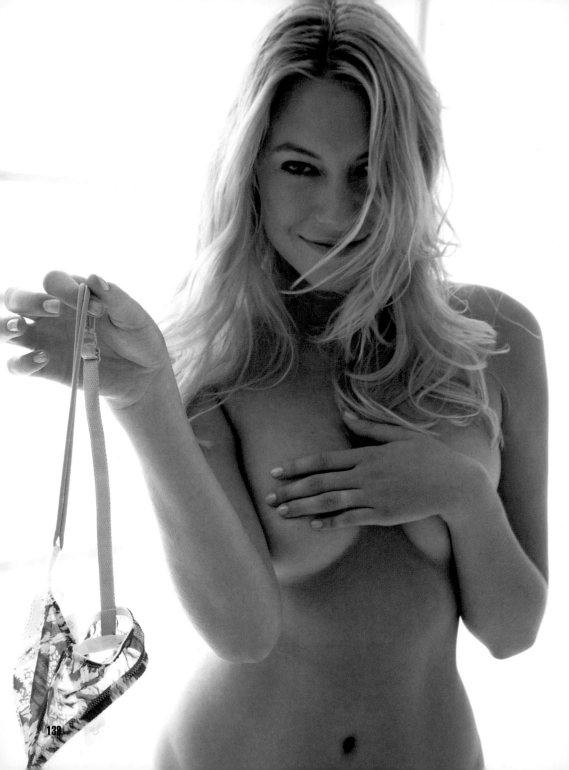

Q: I have a hard time lasting more than 10 minutes during sex. What can I do?

Anytime you feel ready to blow, switch positions or slow down the speed of your thrusting. Jumping to another pose pauses you for a minute and forces your body to relax a bit. Pumping away quickly causes lots of friction, which makes you want to come. So if you slow yourself down, you'll fight that urge. If that doesn't work, try condoms with benzocaine in them—it's a cream that reduces sensation and lets you last longer.

Q: No matter what, my girl can't orgasm during sex. What gives?

If you're expecting her to orgasm during intercourse, many women can't…and there's nothing wrong with that. But her chances will improve if you try positions that provide clitoral stimulation, such as Reach for the Heavens, on page 97, or girl-on-top, which leaves her open for you to manually rub her clitoris. If that doesn't do it, don't push. She'll feel even more self-conscious and be less likely to orgasm. Instead, make sure you help her reach that grand finale through oral sex or by using your hands (try the moves on page 57).

Q: Can women really ejaculate when they climax?

A small amount of fluid is expelled from a woman's urethra when she orgasms. Some researchers believe that at least part of the mystery liquid is produced by the Skene's glands, located on either side of a woman's urethral opening, and that it may be similar in composition to male ejaculate—minus the sperm, of course.

Q: My wife says she feels like she's going to pee when she gets close to a G-spot orgasm, so she makes me stop. Will she?

No. When the G-spot is stimulated, as we explain above, some women emit a small amount of clear fluid from their urethra (don't worry, it's not urine). Because it comes out the same place that pee does, it gives her a very similar feeling and she might assume that's what it is. Tell her you did some research and learned that as long as she pees before the action, she's not actually going to urinate. Simply telling her that may ease her fears enough to relax and let you give her a mind-blowing G-spot orgasm.

Q: She won't let me go down on her. How can I get her to relax?

She's probably nervous that she smells or tastes bad. Or maybe she's worried that she doesn't look "normal" down there. Ease her fears by telling her you love giving her oral and you think every single part of her body—including her V zone—is sexy. Of course, some women simply don't like it, in which case you should stick to manual stimulation or whip out a vibrator and go to town on her.

Q: Would it be bad to take Viagra if I don't need it?

If you have no problems down below, there's absolutely no point in popping that little blue pill. Viagra works by increasing blood flow to your penis, but if everything's already working properly, it doesn't do anything at all—except possibly leave you with a hard-on after you've climaxed. Plus, it's a bad idea (and potentially dangerous) to take meds when they haven't been prescribed to you for a legit medical reason.

Q: My girlfriend tastes a little funky down there. How can I tell her?

You can't…unless you want her to never let you go south again. A variety of things could be causing her to seem less than fresh. Perhaps she had a busy day and was running all over the place and sweating. Also, because of body chemistry, some women take on a different smell or taste down below right before or after their period. Instead of saying anything, suggest taking a shower together as a foreplay move. Or bring a warm, wet washcloth into bed and rub it all over her body, including between her legs. If you're sly about it and rub her in a sexy way, she won't catch on to what you're doing.

Q: I'd like to try anal. How should I bring it up?

One evening when you're lying in bed together, tell her it's something you'd be curious to try. Let her know you'd stop immediately if it didn't feel good, and ask her what she thinks. Not all women are into backdoor lovin', so be okay with her shutting you down. If she *is* willing to try it, put on a condom to prevent spreading bacteria, and use lots of lube—unlike the vagina, the anus isn't self-lubricating. Take it very slowly, and enter her inch by inch. If you're both enjoying yourselves, slowly start thrusting. And if you want to switch to vaginal penetration, make sure you take off the condom so you don't bring all that bacteria into her vagina (it could cause various infections).

SOURCES: AVA CADELL, PHD; HARRY FISCH, MD; SANDOR GARDOS, PHD; IAN KERNER, PHD

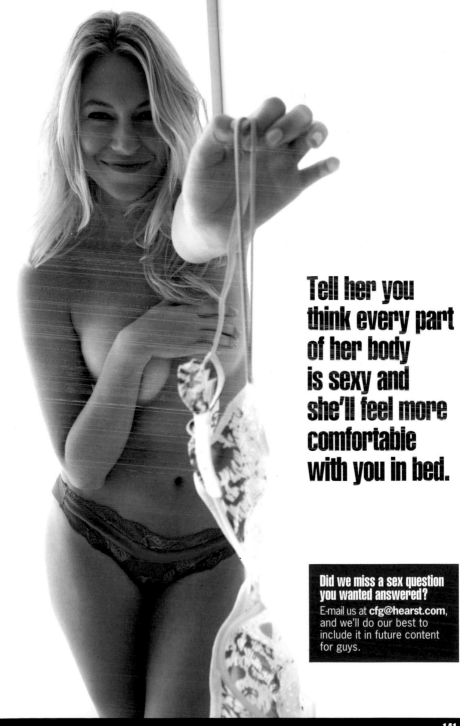

Tell her you think every part of her body is sexy and she'll feel more comfortable with you in bed.

Credits

Cover

Emmet Malström

143

HEARST BOOKS
New York

An Imprint of Sterling Publishing
387 Park Avenue South
New York, NY 10016

COSMOPOLITAN

EDITOR	John Searles
TEXT BY	Bethany Heitman
BOOK DESIGN BY	Peter Perron
COPYEDITED BY	Katy Lindenmuth
EDITOR-IN-CHIEF	Kate White
DESIGN DIRECTOR	Ann P. Kwong

Library of Congress Cataloging-in-Publication Data

Cosmo's satisfy a woman every single time / The editors of *Cosmopolitan* magazine.
    p. cm.
Includes index.
ISBN 978-1-58816-921-1
1. Sex instruction for men. 2. Sexual excitement. 3. Sex. I. *Cosmopolitan* (New York, N.Y. : 1952) II. Title: Satisfy a woman every single time.
  HQ36.C67 2011
  613.9'6081–dc23

                    2011017126

10 9 8 7 6 5 4 3 2 1

Published by Hearst Books
A division of Sterling Publishing Co. Inc.
387 Park Avenue South, New York, NY 10016

Cosmopolitan is a registered trademark of Hearst Communications Inc.

www.cosmopolitan.com

For information about custom editions, special sales, or premium and corporate purchases, please contact Sterling Special Sales Department at 800-805-5489 or specialsales@sterlingpublishing.com.

Distributed in Canada by Sterling Publishing
C/o Canadian Manda Group, 165 Dufferin Street
Toronto, Ontario, Canada M6K 3H6

Distributed in Australia by Capricorn Link (Australia) Pty. Ltd.
P.O. Box 704, Windsor, NSW 2756 Australia

Manufactured in China

Sterling ISBN 978-1-58816-921-1